Childhood Cancer in Britain

Childhood Cancer in Britain
Incidence, survival, mortality

Edited by

Charles Stiller
Senior Research Fellow, Childhood Cancer
Research Group, University of Oxford, UK

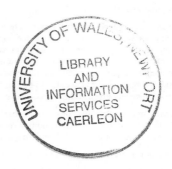
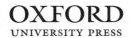

OXFORD
UNIVERSITY PRESS

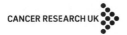

CANCER RESEARCH UK

OXFORD
UNIVERSITY PRESS

Great Clarendon Street, Oxford OX2 6DP

Oxford University Press is a department of the University of Oxford.
It furthers the University's objective of excellence in research, scholarship,
and education by publishing worldwide in

Oxford New York

Auckland Cape Town Dar es Salaam Hong Kong Karachi
Kuala Lumpur Madrid Melbourne Mexico City Nairobi
New Delhi Shanghai Taipei Toronto

With offices in

Argentina Austria Brazil Chile Czech Republic France Greece
Guatemala Hungary Italy Japan South Korea Poland Portugal
Singapore Switzerland Thailand Turkey Ukraine Vietnam

Oxford is a registered trade mark of Oxford University Press
in the UK and in certain other countries

Published in the United States
by Oxford University Press Inc., New York

A catalogue record for this title is available from the British Library

Library of Congress Cataloging in Publication Data

Typeset by Cepha Imaging Pvt Ltd, Bangalore, India
Printed in Great Britain
on acid-free paper by Biddles Ltd., King's Lynn
ISBN 978-0-19-852070-2 (Hbk. : alk.paper)

10 9 8 7 6 5 4 3 2 1

Foreword

There has been enormous progress in the understanding and therapy of children's cancer since 1962, the start of the National Registry of Childhood Tumours, and 1975 when the Childhood Cancer Research Group (CCRG) was founded. The probability of five-year survival of children with cancer has increased dramatically from 28% to 77%; a national organisation responsible for the design, execution and analysis of clinical trials, the United Kingdom Children's Cancer Study Group (UKCCSG) has been established; there is extensive international collaboration in children's cancer trials; care for children with cancer has developed so that over 90% of children are treated at one of the 22 recognised UKCCSG centres; there is a new era which seeks to exploit knowledge of the human genome and newly acquired information on the molecular mechanisms that drive cancer.

These improvements have been possible because there is detailed knowledge of the demographics, including incidence and survival, of childhood cancer provided by the CCRG and the National Registry of Childhood Tumours. Knowledge of the incidence of childhood cancer is vital to the planning of health service provision and the design of research studies, including those relating to the aetiology of childhood cancer. Changes in the incidence of childhood cancer in particular provide important clues as to the aetiology of the disease.

The National Registry of Childhood Tumours is the largest group of cases of childhood cancer in the world and includes over 80,000 cases. The major strengths of the Registry are its population base, the comprehensive ascertainment of cases and the collection and validation of a wide range of data items.

Over the last 30 years the CCRG in Oxford has provided critical information for the development of paediatric oncology, both nationally and internationally, and has been an exemplar for other childhood cancer registries. This book summarises the enormous achievements made by the Group.

The CCRG has had a very close and productive collaboration with the UKCCSG, which is now one of the world's leading co-operative groups for clinical trials in children's cancer. The presentation of changes in survival patterns at the Annual General Meeting of the UKCCSG has provided invaluable insights, which have led the strategic direction of the UKCCSG. Within the UKCCSG, the CCRG has played particularly vital roles in the Clinical Research Governance and the Epidemiology Groups.

Analysis of trends in survival has led to changes in therapeutic approaches, to concentrate efforts on tumour groups associated with the worst survival. These investigations have clearly demonstrated that, at present, the malignancies responsible for the greatest number of deaths from childhood cancer are central nervous system tumours, particularly embryonal tumours and gliomas, neuroblastoma and leukaemia.

There are enormous benefits in the studies of trends in survival carried out by the CCRG. These allow comparison of the effects of different therapeutic approaches in different clinical trials to be demonstrated. Improvements in survival can be linked to time periods when trials are recruiting for specific tumour types, thereby demonstrating the importance of planned successor studies, so that there are no "gaps" in the trial portfolio.

The CCRG has carried out pivotal studies relating the patterns of referral to paediatric oncology centres, the proportion of patients entered on national and international studies, and survival. The Group has provided strong evidence of the benefits of entry into clinical trials, protocol defined treatment and management by multidisciplinary specialist paediatric oncology teams. This has resulted in the international approach towards the entry of children on clinical trials and centralisation of care

Knowledge of the incidence of childhood malignancy in the United Kingdom and comparisons with the incidence in other countries have provided essential data in studies of the epidemiology of childhood cancer. The CCRG has established major and very productive international collaborations with Eurocare and the Automated Childhood Cancer Information System (ACCIS) in Europe. Furthermore, the National Registry of Childhood Tumours complements the Surveillance, Epidemiology and End Results (SEER) Program in North America, thereby allowing important intercontinental comparisons.

The early twenty-first century is an exciting and challenging time for paediatric oncology. Current advances include further developments of clinical trials; the greater understanding of the biology of childhood malignancy which will allow better therapeutic classification and drugs to be designed against targets that drive the malignant process. In addition, there will be further reconfiguration of service delivery and even greater international collaboration.

Important future research led by the CCRG will include more in depth epidemiological studies using case and control data; studies linking malignancy with congenital malformations; monitoring the success of therapeutic approaches and accurately ascertaining the rates of second malignancy, as well as continuing analyses of trends in incidence and survival.

The UKCCSG and its newly formed successor, the Children's Cancer and Leukaemia Group, look forward to an increasingly fruitful relationship with the CCRG. The United Kingdom has in the past benefited greatly by having the invaluable resource of the CCRG; the role of the Group in the future will be even greater.

Professor ADJ Pearson
Cancer Research UK Professor of Paediatric Oncology,
Institute of Cancer Research,
Royal Marsden Hospital
Chair of the United Kingdom Children's Cancer Study Group 2003-2006

Acknowledgements

This book is ostensibly the work of nine named contributors from the Childhood Cancer Research Group (CCRG). In reality, of course, it would not have been possible without the dedicated work of a much larger number of people at the CCRG during the 31 years of its existence and the generous help of many others elsewhere. It is a great pleasure to acknowledge their efforts here, on behalf of myself and my fellow contributors.

We are grateful to all of the following for providing notifications of incident cases of childhood cancer and other information: the English regional cancer registries, now comprising Eastern Cancer Registration and Information Centre, Merseyside and Cheshire Cancer Registry, North Western Cancer Registry, Northern and Yorkshire Cancer Registry and Information Service, Oxford Cancer Intelligence Unit, South and West Cancer Intelligence Service, Thames Cancer Registry, Trent Cancer Registry and West Midlands Cancer Intelligence Unit; the National Cancer Intelligence Centre at the Office for National Statistics (ONS), the Scottish Cancer Registry and the Welsh Cancer Intelligence and Surveillance Unit; Bristol Childhood Cancer Research Registry, Manchester Children's Tumour Registry, Northern Region Young Persons' Malignant Disease Registry, Oxford Region Leukaemia Register, West Midlands Regional Children's Tumour Registry and Yorkshire Specialist Register of Cancer in Children and Young People; the UK Children's Cancer Study Group (UKCCSG); the Childhood Leukaemia Working Party and the Clinical Trial Service Unit. Death notifications have been supplied by ONS (for England and Wales) and the General Register Office (Scotland). Many of the above organizations have undergone changes of name or amalgamation during the past decades. This acknowledgement should be understood to encompass all previous incarnations of these bodies and their constituents that have contributed data to the National Registry of Childhood Tumours (NRCT), and in many cases initially to the Oxford Survey of Childhood Cancers (OSCC). We are grateful to the NHS Central Registers at Southport and Dumfries (formerly Edinburgh) for flagging tens of thousands of children from the NRCT. Without this extremely accurate and efficient system, follow-up on this scale would be prohibitively time-consuming and costly, and undoubtedly less complete. We also thank the many members of the UKCCSG and other consultants and general practitioners who have provided information about patients under their care.

It would take too much space to acknowledge the contributions of every individual at the CCRG by name, but the roles of the following people have been especially important: the CCRG's founding Director, Gerald Draper, and his successor, Mike Murphy; Registry Supervisors Betty Roberts, Maureen Allen and Anita Bayne, Medical Research Officers Elizabeth Lennox, Bridget Caplan and Liz Eatock, Registry Assistants Anita Rich and Martin King and Computing Assistant Jean Williams and their predecessors for their hard work and attention to detail in maintaining the NRCT; Barbara Sanders for collecting much detailed information, especially relating to children with retinoblastoma; Tim Vincent for much work on geographical coding and birth records which, while not directly used in this volume, has played an important part in maintaining data quality, and for ensuring that the most up-to-date estimates of population at risk were available for the incidence and mortality analyses; Pat Brownbill and her colleagues and predecessors for development and maintenance of the computing system on which we all depend. Mike Hawkins and his colleagues, initially at the CCRG and now at the Centre for Childhood Cancer Survivor Studies, University of Birmingham, have contributed much valuable information, especially on follow-up and multiple tumours. We thank Gerald Draper and John Bithell for advice on statistical methods and the interpretation of results in Chapter 4. I am also personally indebted to John Bithell, whose suggestion that I analyse data from the OSCC as a postgraduate student initiated me into childhood cancer epidemiology. Particular thanks are due to Janette King for typing a large part of the text and tables and for assembling these and everybody else's contributions in the appropriate format, and for maintaining the CCRG's bibliographic database. Most of the figures were produced by authors of the chapters in which they appear, but Pat Brownbill and Janette King produced several of the graphs for Chapter 5.

In addition to providing information on cases of childhood cancer, many individuals and organizations have over the years asked us a great many questions on the statistics of childhood cancer. We are grateful to all those whose queries have suggested ways of looking at the data or particular groups of cases that were worthy of analysis.

I am very grateful to Helen Liepman, Georgia Pinteau and Clare Caruana at Oxford University Press for their patient encouragement throughout this project.

Financial support for statistical analyses was provided by Cancer Research UK. The CCRG receives funding from the Department of Health and the Scottish Ministers. The views expressed in the publication are those of the authors and not necessarily those of the Department of Health and the Scottish Ministers.

Contents

Abbreviations

AAPC	Average annual percent change	ICD	International Classification of Diseases
ACC	Adrenocortical carcinoma	ICD-O	International Classification of Diseases for Oncology
ACCIS	Automated Childhood Cancer Information System	ICD-O-2	International Classification of Diseases for Oncology, Second Edition
ALCL	Anaplastic large cell lymphoma		
ALL	Acute lymphoblastic leukaemia	ICD-O-3	International Classification of Diseases for Oncology, Third Edition
AML	Acute myeloid leukaemia		
ASR	Age-standardized rate	IICC	International Incidence of Childhood Cancer (Volume One, Volume Two)
ATRT	Atypical teratoid rhabdoid tumour	(-1, -2)	
BCC	Basal cell carcinoma	ISD	Information and Statistics Division (of the Scottish Health Service)
BCCSS	British Childhood Cancer Survivor Study		
		JMML	Juvenile myelomonocytic leukaemia
BFM	Berlin–Frankfurt–Münster	MDS	Myelodysplastic syndrome
CBTRUS	Central Brain Tumor Registry of the United States	MFH	Malignant fibrous histiocytoma
		MOTNAC	Manual of Tumor Nomenclature and Coding
CCRG	Childhood Cancer Research Group		
CCSS	Childhood Cancer Survivor Study	MPNST	Malignant peripheral nerve sheath tumour
CI	(95%) confidence interval		
CLWP	Childhood Leukaemia Working Party	MRC	Medical Research Council
CML	Chronic myeloid leukaemia	MRI	Magnetic resonance imaging
CMML	Chronic myelomonocytic leukaemia	NHL	Non-Hodgkin lymphoma
CNS	Central nervous system	NHSCR	National Health Service Central Registers
COMARE	Committee on Medical Aspects of Radiation in the Environment		
		NOS	Not otherwise specified
CT	Computed tomography	NRCT	National Registry of Childhood Tumours
DCO	Death certificate only		
DFSP	Dermatofibrosarcoma protuberans	NWTS	National Wilms Tumor Study
DNET	Dysembryoplastic neuroepithelial tumour	ONS	Office for National Statistics
		OPCS	Office of Population Censuses and Surveys
DSRCT	Desmoplastic small round cell tumour		
EMF	Electromagnetic fields	PIAG	Patient Information Advisory Group
ENSG	European Neuroblastoma Study Group	PNET	Primitive neuroectodermal tumour
ESFT	Ewing sarcoma family of tumours	pPNET	Peripheral primitive neuroectodermal tumour
FAB	French–American–British		
GRO(S)	General Register Office (Scotland)	SEER	Surveillance, Epidemiology, and End Results
HCC	Hepatocellular carcinoma		
HIV	Human immunodeficiency virus	SIOP	Société Internationale d'Oncologie Pédiatrique (International Society of Paediatric Oncology)
ICCC	International Classification of Childhood Cancer		
		UKCCSG	United Kingdom Children's Cancer Study Group
ICCC-3	International Classification of Childhood Cancer, Third Edition		

Contributors

Anita M Bayne
Registry Supervisor,
Childhood Cancer Research Group,
University of Oxford, UK

Pat A Brownbill
I.T. Manager,
Childhood Cancer Research Group,
University of Oxford, UK

Kathryn Bunch
Research Officer,
Childhood Cancer Research Group,
University of Oxford, UK

Gerald Draper
Honorary Senior Research Fellow,
Childhood Cancer Research Group,
University of Oxford, UK

Elizabeth M Eatock
Medical Research Officer,
Childhood Cancer Research Group,
University of Oxford, UK

Mary E Kroll
Statistician,
Childhood Cancer Research Group,
University of Oxford, UK

Michael Murphy
Consultant Epidemiologist & Director,
Childhood Cancer Research Group,
University of Oxford, UK

Charles A Stiller
Senior Research Fellow,
Childhood Cancer Research Group,
University of Oxford, UK

Tim J Vincent
Childhood Cancer Research Group,
University of Oxford, UK

Chapter 1

Introduction

GJ Draper

The material presented in this volume is based on records in the National Registry of Childhood Tumours (NRCT) maintained by the Childhood Cancer Research Group (CCRG).

Childhood tumours, defined here (as is usual) as tumours occurring before the age of 15 years, represent only about 1 in 200 cases of cancer occurring in the UK, but are the subject of great public concern. There is a large ongoing research effort into both the causes and the treatment of these conditions. The NRCT is a major source of data for this work and for information about the occurrence and consequences of childhood cancer.

In this chapter, we describe briefly the origins and functions of the CCRG and the NRCT and relate these to the development of cancer registration, and particularly children's cancer registration, in the UK. Methodological aspects of cancer registration in relation to the NRCT are described in Chapter 2. Analyses of the NRCT data are presented in Chapters 3–6. A review of the uses of the data is given in Chapter 7.

1.1 Historical developments

1.1.1 History of the Childhood Cancer Research Group

Between 1956 and 1973, a nationwide case-control study of children with cancer (the Oxford Survey of Childhood Cancers (OSCC)), designed to investigate a variety of possible aetiological factors, was carried out at the Department of Social Medicine at Oxford under the direction of the late Dr Alice Stewart, Reader in Social Medicine (Stewart *et al.*, 1958). This study originally included children who died of cancer from 1953 onwards, notifications being received through death certificates. The data collection was later extended so that registrations of cancer incidence for children diagnosed from 1962 onwards were also obtained; it then became possible to carry out analyses of incidence and survival rates.

In 1973, the Department of Health Standing Medical Advisory Committee (SMAC) Sub-Committee on Cancer set up a working party on childhood tumour registration. This working party reported in 1974 and, as a result of its recommendations, the CCRG was established in April 1975. The registration and death certificate data collected as part of the extended OSCC formed the basis for what was to become the NRCT.

The SMAC Working Party recommended that the group should:

(I) maintain a register of childhood tumours similar to the National Cancer Registration Scheme (which covers all age groups) but with additional information, and that statistical data in more detail than that provided by the Office of Population Censuses and Surveys (OPCS) (now the Office for National Statistics (ONS)) should be provided;

(II) provide information for the planning and monitoring of health care services;

(III) establish standards for the outcome of treatment;

(IV) carry out epidemiological studies;

(V) assist with clinical trials;

(VI) set up and advise on standards for recording, documentation, classification and nomenclature; and

(VII) give access to the registry to *bona fide* research workers.

Since its establishment, the Group has been a part of the University of Oxford and is funded mainly by the Department of Health and the Scottish Executive, with project grants from charities such as the Cancer Research Campaign (now Cancer Research UK), the Leukaemia Research Fund, the Kay Kendall Leukaemia Fund, the Retinoblastoma Society (now the Childhood Eye Cancer Trust) and Children with Leukaemia.

1.1.2 The development of cancer registration and of childhood cancer registries in the UK

Cancer registration in the UK started in the 1920s in several parts of the country, with the commencement of radium treatment, in order to follow the outcome of treated patients. Later the objectives became broader. By 1959, cancer registration was national in Scotland and, by 1962, it was national in England and Wales. It was, and remains, a voluntary rather than statutory system. A standardized minimum data set has evolved and the coding and classification of cancers has followed international standards, namely the International Classification of Diseases and the International Classification of Diseases for Oncology (World Health Organization, 2000). Most of the analyses and reports from cancer registries deal mainly with adult cancers and use a site-based system for classifying tumours. Childhood tumours are more naturally classified by histological type of tumour. The rarity of childhood tumours (only 1 in 200 of the cancer cases occurring in the UK), and the fact that the types of cancer are often different from those occurring in adults, mean that their classification requires specialist knowledge. Furthermore, it is often useful to collect information additional to that available for the generality of adult cases. Although childhood cases form only a small proportion of total cancer cases, cancer is an important cause of morbidity and mortality in childhood and the need for specialized registries of childhood tumours and for analyses based on these has been recognized for some decades. Such specialized registries also reflect the particular need for follow-up among childhood cancer survivors and the desirability of monitoring their progress in collaboration with their clinical consultants.

1.1.3 The Manchester Children's Tumour Registry

The first childhood tumour registry in the world, the Manchester Children's Tumour Registry, covering a population of about one million children aged 0–14 years in north-west

England, was set up in 1953 (Birch, 1988). This registry still exists. The registry has a high level of completeness of ascertainment of cases, and diagnoses are subject to detailed pathological review. Information from this registry has formed the basis for a series of research papers.

1.1.4 Childhood tumour registries – nationally and internationally

There are now several childhood tumour registries covering various regions of the UK (see Chapter 2), and many elsewhere, covering complete countries or regions within them. Information on the occurrence of childhood cancer in many parts of the world has been published in the two volumes, *International Incidence of Childhood Cancer*, (Parkin *et al.*, 1988b, 1998). These volumes include data from both specialized paediatric cancer registries and general cancer registries.

1.1.5 The National Registry of Childhood Tumours

The first childhood tumour registry having national coverage was the National Registry of Childhood Tumours (NRCT). This is a population-based registry of cancers diagnosed at ages 0–14 years from 1962 onwards in residents of England, Scotland and Wales. The NRCT also includes data for Northern Ireland from 1993, so that coverage is now complete for the UK. (The present volume does not include data from Northern Ireland.) The registry also includes mortality data from 1953 onwards for England, Wales and Scotland. (The definition of deaths to be included has varied in terms of age and diagnostic categories.) Before the registry was set up there had been, in effect, a register of all deaths from childhood cancer in England, Scotland and Wales in the form of records collected in the course of a national case-control study (the OSCC) carried out by Dr Alice Stewart, referred to above. In the latter years of this research project, records relating to children notified to the national cancer registration scheme were also collected. The construction of manual indexes and computer files of registration and death certificate data for the OSCC produced the basis for the NRCT. The registry now has a high level of ascertainment based on multiple sources of information – see Chapter 2. Members of the CCRG have published a large series of research papers using these data, and the Registry has also been used for national and international studies carried out by, or in collaboration with, other research workers and clinicians.

1.2 Objectives of the analyses presented in this volume

We present here a series of analyses of the registry data; these analyses are based on the largest national series of cases of childhood cancer ever published. The scope of this volume is similar to that of the previously published analyses of incidence and survival from the United States Surveillance, Epidemiology and End Results (SEER) Program (Ries *et al.*, 1999). Our objective is to present descriptive data and analyses from the NRCT as a reference source for clinicians, epidemiologists, health administrators and others needing information about cancer in children. These data and analyses are presented in Chapters 3–6, and described briefly below.

1.2.1 **Incidence rates and trends in incidence**

Chapter 3, on incidence rates, is relevant to the planning of health service provision and also to the design of research studies on the aetiology of childhood cancers. It is also, when combined with similar data from other countries, of direct value in attempting to identify aetiological factors. The information on age distributions – which we believe to be the most detailed ever published – gives some insight, particularly when combined with information on the types of cell involved, into the likely times of initiation of the various tumour types, and hence into questions of aetiology. There are clear similarities and differences in the distributions for different diagnostic groups, which may give clues to corresponding similarities and differences in aetiological factors and times of initiation.

Chapter 4, on trends in incidence, is relevant to frequently raised questions about whether increasing levels of environmental pollutants, or changes in other possibly relevant aetiological factors, lead to changes in rates of childhood cancer. Since changes in many environmental factors may occur simultaneously, it is unlikely that such data will by themselves provide strong evidence about aetiology. The exception might be if the sudden introduction or removal of a putative aetiological agent were to be followed by a change in incidence. We emphasize that, before aetiological inferences can be made, it is essential to consider other, non-causal, reasons for apparent changes in incidence: these include changes in the proportions of cases notified to the registry, changes in the proportions of cases correctly diagnosed, and changes in systems of diagnostic classification. Possible artefacts are discussed in detail in Chapter 4.

1.2.2 **Survival and mortality rates**

Chapter 5, on survival and trends in survival, shows where progress has been made and the extent to which the well-recognized successes in specialist centres are reflected nationally (though in the UK the great majority of children are now in fact treated in specialist centres and expertise is shared between these centres). Again, these data are relevant for planning purposes, in showing the number of patients on long-term follow-up and requiring surveillance.

Chapter 6, on mortality, is another way of demonstrating the progress made in the treatment of childhood cancer, though mortality rates are of course dependent on both incidence and survival rates.

1.3 **Wider objectives of the Registry**

In common with other cancer registries, the NRCT is used as the basis for a large number of research studies, some carried out by members of the Childhood Cancer Research Group (CCRG), possibly in collaboration with others outside the group, and some carried out by external research workers. In Chapter 7, we give an indication of the range of uses of the Registry data. Some of these uses depend on aspects of the Registry data not analysed in the present volume but discussed in Chapter 7, for instance the fact that a large proportion of the records have been combined with information from birth records: this opens up possibilities for other aetiological analyses. Again, the availability of identifying information makes it possible, subject to very stringent conditions designed to protect confidentiality, to carry out a variety of record linkage studies. We hope that as a result of publication of the analyses presented here other research workers, clinicians and administrators will become aware of the potential of the Registry for research and administrative purposes and will make use of the data both directly and as a starting point for further work.

Chapter 2

Methods

TJ Vincent, AM Bayne, PA Brownbill and CA Stiller

2.1 The National Registry of Childhood Tumours

One of the main functions of the Childhood Cancer Research Group is to maintain the population-based National Registry of Childhood Tumours (NRCT) covering cases diagnosed at ages 0–14 years in England, Wales and Scotland. About 1 in 500 children develop some form of cancer before their 15th birthday. This represents approximately 1500 new cases diagnosed each year. The NRCT is the largest register of childhood cancer in the world and in 2006 includes nearly 80,000 cases. The success of the registry depends upon the comprehensive ascertainment of cases and the collection and validation of a wide range of data items. This is facilitated by the collaboration of a number of other organizations. The registry does not itself engage in active case-finding.

2.2 Sources of ascertainment

2.2.1 Cancer registries

Cancer registration in England is carried out by a network of population-based regional registries, and coverage has been national since 1962. Registration is coordinated by the Office for National Statistics (ONS), who maintain a national cancer registry covering all age groups. Until devolution in 1999, cancer registration in Wales was included as part of the England and Wales regional cancer registration system with data coordinated and published by ONS. Since devolution, Wales has a distinct national cancer registry. In Scotland, a cancer registration system has been in operation since 1959. This was originally based on five regional registries, and coordinated by the Information and Statistics Division (ISD) of the Scottish Health Service, but since 1997 there has been a single, national registry for the whole of Scotland. The first cancer registry for Northern Ireland was established in 1959 and was re-established in 1994 based at Queen's University of Belfast. Copies of all registrations from 1962 onwards relating to children aged under 15 years have been sent to the NRCT by ONS, ISD and the cancer registries.

There are also several specialist children's tumour registries in various parts of Britain which register cases occurring in their own localities and notify these to the NRCT. These include the Manchester Children's Tumour Registry (Birch, 1988), the Northern Region Young Persons' Malignant Disease Registry (Cotterill *et al.*, 2000b), the West Midlands Regional Children's Tumour Registry (Parkes *et al.*, 1997) and the Yorkshire Specialist Register of Cancer in Children and Young People (McKinney *et al.*, 1998). Cases have also been ascertained from a ten-year population-based study of childhood cancer in south-west England (Foreman *et al.*, 1994), recently reactivated as the Bristol Childhood Cancer Research Registry, and from the Oxford Region Leukaemia Register (Stiller *et al.*, 1999).

A regular exchange and validation of data takes place between the NRCT and the various regional and national registries. Cancer is not a legally notifiable disease, so reporting to the registries is voluntary. Methods and completeness of ascertainment of cases have varied with time and between registries. Commonly used sources have included hospital case notes and diagnostic indexes, computerized in-patient records, pathology departments and death certificates and general practitioner notes.

2.2.2 The Children's Cancer and Leukaemia Group and its predecessors

The Childhood Leukaemia Working Party (CLWP) has organized a series of clinical trials for more than 35 years. For many years it operated under the auspices of the Medical Research Council (MRC) but it is now part of the National Cancer Research Institute. Notification of children entered in the leukaemia trials since 1970 have been supplied to the CCRG, initially by the MRC Leukaemia Trials Office and subsequently by the Clinical Trial Service Unit at Oxford.

The United Kingdom Children's Cancer Study Group (UKCCSG) was set up in 1977 as the national organization for paediatric oncologists and other clinicians and scientists with a particular interest in childhood cancer (UKCCSG, 2002). Since then it has expanded to a maximum of 22 UKCCSG centres, responsible for the care of nearly all children presenting with malignant disease in the UK and Eire. From the outset, the UKCCSG has maintained a register of the children with cancer under the care of its members. The UKCCSG coordinates clinical trials for all the major types of childhood cancer except leukaemia. The UKCCSG data centre in Leicester provides the NRCT with copies of notifications to the register of patients and information on children entered into trials. The CCRG is responsible for the routine follow-up of patients in the register and collaborates in the production of the UKCCSG annual Scientific Reports. These reports present analyses of the patterns of referral to paediatric oncology centres, the survival rates of UKCCSG patients and the proportions of UKCCSG patients who are entered in national and international clinical trials and studies.

In August 2006, the UKCCSG and CLWP merged under the title of Children's Cancer and Leukaemia Group.

2.2.3 Death certification

In the very early years for which cancer data were collected, death certification was the principal source of ascertainment of cases. At this time survival rates were very low, hence mortality for some diagnoses, particularly leukaemia, would have been a close approximation to incidence. Survival rates have since improved dramatically, and with the establishment of the national cancer registration system in 1962 and the UKCCSG in 1977, the number of cases now ascertained solely from death certification is small. Copies of death certificates for all deaths occurring before the age of 20 years with a neoplasm coded as the underlying cause are sent to the CCRG by ONS (for England and Wales) and by the General Register Office (GRO) (for Scotland).

2.3 Completeness of ascertainment

The completeness of ascertainment has obviously varied over time and between registries but with notifications often being received from more than one source it is believed that ascertainment is now almost complete. Table 2.1 shows the numbers of cases, diagnosed between specified years, that were notified from different sources. From the early 1970s over 97% were picked up by the cancer registration system and an ever increasing proportion of cases are notified to the NRCT by more than one source. The steady decline in the number of cases being notified from death certificates is a result of dramatic improvements in treatment and survival over the last 40 years. For leukaemia, which is the largest single group of cases, accounting for about one-third of all childhood cancers in the UK, it has been estimated that the NRCT is 99% complete (based on the assumption of independence of the various sources) (Stiller *et al.*, 1991b). A very high degree of ascertainment is essential to having any confidence in analyses of incidence, survival and mortality such as those presented in the subsequent chapters of this book.

2.4 Data collection and validation

The NRCT collects much more information and in particular more detailed diagnostic data than are available in the general cancer registration system. The NRCT is able to do this partly because it is concentrating on only a very small proportion of the total number of cancer cases occurring in the population, and partly because data are collected from a greater number of sources. Each of these provides a variety of data items, many of which can be cross-checked and computer validated. The histological diagnosis and date of diagnosis, together with initial treatment, follow-up and other clinical data, are verified and amended where appropriate using the records held by the hospitals at which the children were treated, by their general practitioners or by the organizers of clinical trials. In addition, the diagnoses for the great majority of children in the regional children's tumour registries are centrally reviewed and their records checked against those in the NRCT.

The CCRG also collates additional information which facilitates other types of study not presented in this volume. Information from birth registration documents is collected allowing the study of factors such as address and parental occupation at the time of birth. Information relating to subsequent primary tumours occurring in the same individual is important in the consideration of some genetic factors and possible side-effects of the treatment of the initial malignancy. Other genetic studies require the collection of information on the siblings of affected children, and in some instances on other family members.

2.5 Follow-up and NHS central registers

Details of all children who survive for at least five years after diagnosis are sent to the National Health Service Central Registers (NHSCR) in Southport and Edinburgh. These individuals are identified in the Register and a flag (marker label) attached to their record.

Table 2.1 Sources of notification for children in the NRCT diagnosed with a malignant disease and normally resident in England, Wales or Scotland

Source	1966–70 Number (%)	1971–75 Number (%)	1976–80 Number (%)	1981–85 Number (%)	1986–90 Number (%)	1991–95 Number (%)	1996–2000 Number (%)	1991–2000 Number (%)
Total cases	6668 (100)	6902 (100)	6596 (100)	6131 (100)	6568 (100)	7252 (100)	7407 (100)	14,659 (100)
National and regional cancer registries	6121 (91.8)	6727 (97.5)	6486 (98.3)	6057 (98.8)	6484 (98.7)	7047 (97.2)	7232 (97.6)	14,279 (97.4)
UKCCSG	3 (0.04)	22 (0.32)	2465 (37.4)	4085 (66.6)	4973 (75.7)	6201 (85.5)	6722 (90.8)	12,923 (88.2)
Leukaemia trials	61 (0.91)	1030 (14.9)	1223 (18.5)	1124 (18.3)	1439 (21.9)	1837 (25.3)	1948 (26.3)	3785 (25.8)
Death certificate	4975 (74.6)	4315 (62.5)	3435 (52.1)	2526 (41.2)	2327 (35.4)	2115 (29.2)	1770 (23.9)	3885 (26.5)
All 4 sources	0 (0.00)	3 (0.04)	272 (4.12)	340 (5.55)	394 (6.00)	423 (5.83)	370 (5.00)	793 (5.41)
Any 3 sources	36 (0.54)	582 (8.43)	1567 (23.8)	1974 (32.2)	2325 (35.4)	2775 (38.3)	2783 (37.6)	5558 (37.9)
Any 2 sources	4420 (66.3)	4019 (58.2)	3063 (46.4)	2693 (43.9)	2823 (43.0)	3129 (43.1)	3589 (48.5)	6718 (45.8)
Any 1 source	2212 (33.2)	2298 (33.3)	1694 (25.7)	1124 (18.3)	1026 (15.6)	925 (12.8)	665 (8.98)	1590 (10.8)

This flag signifies that the NRCT is to be notified of any future cancer registration or death certificate received by NHSCR relating to this individual. Together with notifications of embarkations (resulting in loss to follow-up when a person emigrates), these data are used to calculate survival rates and as a source of ascertainment of subsequent primary neoplasms. As Table 2.2 shows, only a very small proportion of cases are lost to follow-up (less than 1% for the period 1991–2000).

2.6 Coding and classification of diagnoses

The distinctive pathological nature of most childhood cancers has long been recognized. The most common forms of cancer in children are leukaemias (about one-third of cases) and neoplasms of the brain and spinal cord (about one-quarter), whereas the cancers most common in adults (carcinomas of lung, female breast, stomach, large bowel and prostate) are extremely rare. Cancers in children exhibit great histological diversity, and some types of childhood tumour can arise in a wide variety of anatomical sites. Consequently, it is essential for data on childhood tumours to be recorded in a way that preserves information about their histology as well as their primary sites. The diagnoses of case children in the Oxford Survey of Childhood Cancers, which provided the initial data set for the NRCT (see Chapter 1), were coded according to a specially developed system that included detailed information on both primary site and histological type. Since the mid-1970s, the topography and morphology of neoplasms in the NRCT have been coded according to successive standard international systems, namely the *Manual of Tumour Nomenclature and Coding* (MOTNAC) (American Cancer Society, 1968) and the first and second editions of the *International Classification of Diseases for Oncology* (ICD-O) (World Health Organization, 1976, 1990). The NRCT will convert to the third edition of ICD-O (World Health Organization 2000) in the near future; meanwhile, ICD-O-3 codes have been adopted for entities not included in ICD-O-2. In addition to the ICD-O codes, the analyses in this volume also make use of data on immunophenotype (for lymphoid neoplasms), French–American–British subtype (for acute myeloid leukaemia) and laterality (for retinoblastoma and renal tumours).

Cancer registries covering all age groups routinely collect information on morphology, but cancer incidence data for adults are still generally tabulated according to the International Classification of Diseases (ICD), in which cancers other than leukaemias, lymphomas, cutaneous melanomas and, most recently, mesothelioma and Kaposi sarcoma are grouped by site of origin (Parkin *et al.*, 2002). By contrast, about 30 years ago, data from the Third National Cancer Survey in the United States (Young and Miller, 1975) and from the NRCT and the Manchester Children's Tumour Registry in Britain (Draper *et al.*, 1982) were already presented according to hierarchical diagnostic classifications in which histological type played an important part. The classification in the latter study was the first in which the diagnostic categories were defined explicitly in terms of a standard coding system, namely MOTNAC. The first internationally accepted classification for childhood cancer was devised by Birch and Marsden (1987). In this scheme there were 12 diagnostic groups, most of which were partitioned into several subgroups.

Table 2.2 Follow-up status for children in the NRCT diagnosed with a malignant disease and normally resident in England, Wales or Scotland

Status	1966–70 Number (%)	1971–75 Number (%)	1976–80 Number (%)	1981–85 Number (%)	1986–90 Number (%)	1991–95 Number (%)	1996–2000 Number (%)	1991–2000 Number (%)
Total cases	6668 (100)	6902 (100)	6596 (100)	6131 (100)	6568 (100)	7252 (100)	7407 (100)	14,659 (100)
With follow-up (DC and/or flag)	6580 (98.7)	6795 (98.4)	6494 (98.5)	6037 (98.5)	6449 (98.2)	7176 (99.0)	7334 (99.0)	14,510 (99.0)
Emigrated	74 (1.11)	90 (1.30)	81 (1.23)	68 (1.11)	63 (0.96)	35 (0.48)	46 (0.62)	81 (0.55)
Untraced at NHSCR	9 (0.13)	16 (0.23)	20 (0.30)	22 (0.36)	42 (0.64)	35 (0.48)	23 (0.31)	58 (0.40)
No DC, not yet sent for flagging	5 (0.07)	1 (0.01)	1 (0.02)	4 (0.07)	14 (0.21)	6 (0.08)	4 (.05)	10 (0.07)

The groups and subgroups were defined according to codes for topography and morphology in the first edition of the ICD-O. This classification was used in the first volume of *International Incidence of Childhood Cancer* (IICC) (Parkin *et al.*, 1988b) and was rapidly accepted as a worldwide standard. Subsequently the International Classification of Childhood Cancer (ICCC) (Kramárová and Stiller, 1996) was constructed, with diagnostic categories defined by the codes in ICD-O-2. Its guiding principles were to take account of scientific developments while preserving the underlying concepts and hierarchical structure of the Birch and Marsden classification. The ICCC was used in the second volume of IICC (Parkin *et al.*, 1998) and, as with its predecessor, soon became the standard international classification for the presentation of incidence and survival data on childhood cancer (Ries *et al.*, 1999; Capocaccia *et al.*, 2001; Steliarova-Foucher *et al.*, 2004). Most recently, the ICCC, third edition (ICCC-3) (Steliarova-Foucher *et al.*, 2005b) was developed, based on the codes in ICD-O-3. Again, the aim was to produce an up-to-date classification that nevertheless had as much continuity as possible with its predecessors. In particular, it conformed to internationally accepted classifications of the pathology and genetics of neoplasms, including such volumes as had been published in the ongoing series *WHO Classification of Tumours*. It carried forward the basic structure of main diagnostic groups and subgroups but, in addition, selected subgroups were further classified into divisions. The groups, subgroups and divisions within the classification are given below:

I Leukaemias, myeloproliferative diseases and myelodysplastic diseases
  a. Lymphoid leukaemias
    1. Precursor cell leukaemias
    2. Mature B-cell leukaemias
    3. Mature T-cell and NK cell leukaemias
    4. Lymphoid leukaemia, NOS
  b. Acute myeloid leukaemias
  c. Chronic myeloproliferative diseases
  d. Myelodysplastic syndrome and other myeloproliferative diseases
  e. Unspecified and other specified leukaemias
II Lymphomas and reticuloendothelial neoplasms
  a. Hodgkin lymphomas
  b. Non-Hodgkin lymphomas (except Burkitt lymphoma)
    1. Precursor cell lymphomas
    2. Mature B-cell lymphomas (except Burkitt lymphoma)
    3. Mature T-cell and NK cell lymphomas
    4. Non-Hodgkin lymphomas, NOS
  c. Burkitt lymphoma
  d. Miscellaneous lymphoreticular neoplasms
  e. Unspecified lymphomas

III Central nervous system and miscellaneous intracranial and intraspinal neoplasms
  a. Ependymomas and choroid plexus tumour
    1. Ependymomas
    2. Choroid plexus tumour
  b. Astrocytomas
  c. Intracranial and intraspinal embryonal tumours
    1. Medulloblastomas
    2. Primitive neuroectodermal tumours (PNETs)
    3. Medulloepithelioma
    4. Atypical teratoid/rhabdoid tumour
  d. Other gliomas
    1. Oligodendrogliomas
    2. Mixed and unspecified gliomas
    3. Neuroepithelial glial tumours of uncertain origin
  e. Other specified intracranial and intraspinal neoplasms
    1. Pituitary adenomas and carcinomas
    2. Tumours of the sellar region (craniopharyngiomas)
    3. Pineal parenchymal tumours
    4. Neuronal and mixed neuronal–glial tumours
    5. Meningiomas
  f. Unspecified intracranial and intraspinal neoplasms
IV Neuroblastoma and other peripheral nervous cell tumours
  a. Neuroblastoma and ganglioneuroblastoma
  b. Other peripheral nervous cell tumours
V Retinoblastoma
VI Renal tumours
  a. Nephroblastoma and other nonepithelial renal tumours
    1. Nephroblastoma
    2. Rhabdoid renal tumour
    3. Kidney sarcomas
    4. Peripheral neuroectodermal tumour (pPNET) of kidney
  b. Renal carcinomas
  c. Unspecified malignant renal tumours
VII Hepatic tumours
  a. Hepatoblastoma
  b. Hepatic carcinomas
  c. Unspecified malignant hepatic tumours

VIII Malignant bone tumours
  a. Osteosarcomas
  b. Chondrosarcomas
  c. Ewing tumour and related sarcomas of bone
    1. Ewing tumour and Askin tumour of bone
    2. Peripheral neuroectodermal tumour (pPNET) of bone
  d. Other specified malignant bone tumours
    1. Malignant fibrous neoplasms of bone
    2. Malignant chordomas
    3. Odontogenic malignant tumours
    4. Miscellaneous malignant bone tumours
  e. Unspecified malignant bone tumours

IX Soft tissue and other extraosseous sarcomas
  a. Rhabdomyosarcomas
  b. Fibrosarcomas, peripheral nerve sheath tumours and other fibrous neoplasms
    1. Fibroblastic and myofibroblastic tumours
    2. Nerve sheath tumours
    3. Other fibromatous neoplasms
  c. Kaposi sarcoma
  d. Other specified soft tissue sarcomas
    1. Ewing tumour and Askin tumour of soft tissue
    2. Peripheral neuroectodermal tumour (pPNET) of soft tissue
    3. Extrarenal rhabdoid tumour
    4. Liposarcomas
    5. Fibrohistiocytic tumours
    6. Leiomyosarcomas
    7. Synovial sarcomas
    8. Blood vessel tumours
    9. Osseous and chondromatous neoplasms of soft tissue
    10. Alveolar soft parts sarcoma
    11. Miscellaneous soft tissue sarcomas
  e. Unspecified soft tissue sarcomas

X Germ cell tumours, trophoblastic tumours and neoplasms of gonads
  a. Intracranial and intraspinal germ cell tumours
    1. Intracranial and intraspinal germinomas
    2. Intracranial and intraspinal teratomas
    3. Intracranial and intraspinal embryonal carcinomas

4. Intracranial and intraspinal yolk sac tumour

5. Intracranial and intraspinal choriocarcinoma

6. Intracranial and intraspinal tumours of mixed forms

b. Malignant extracranial and extragonadal germ cell tumours

1. Malignant germinomas of extracranial and extragonadal sites

2. Malignant teratomas of extracranial and extragonadal sites

3. Embryonal carcinomas of extracranial and extragonadal sites

4. Yolk sac tumour of extracranial and extragonadal sites

5. Choriocarcinomas of extracranial and extragonadal sites

6. Other and unspecified malignant mixed germ cell tumours of extracranial and extragonadal sites

c. Malignant gonadal germ cell tumours

1. Malignant gonadal germinomas

2. Malignant gonadal teratomas

3. Gonadal embryonal carcinomas

4. Gonadal yolk sac tumour

5. Gonadal choriocarcinoma

6. Malignant gonadal tumours of mixed forms

7. Malignant gonadal gonadoblastoma

d. Gonadal carcinomas

e. Other and unspecified malignant gonadal tumours

XI Other malignant epithelial neoplasms and malignant melanomas

a. Adrenocortical carcinomas

b. Thyroid carcinomas

c. Nasopharyngeal carcinomas

d. Malignant melanomas

e. Skin carcinomas

f. Other and unspecified carcinomas

1. Carcinomas of salivary glands

2. Carcinomas of colon and rectum

3. Carcinomas of appendix

4. Carcinomas of lung

5. Carcinomas of thymus

6. Carcinomas of breast

7. Carcinomas of cervix uteri

8. Carcinomas of bladder

9. Carcinomas of eye

10. Carcinomas of other specified sites

11. Carcinomas of unspecified site

XII Other and unspecified malignant neoplasms

    a. Other specified malignant tumours

        1. Gastrointestinal stromal tumour

        2. Pancreatoblastoma

        3. Pulmonary blastoma and pleuropulmonary blastoma

        4. Other complex mixed and stromal neoplasms

        5. Mesothelioma

        6. Other specified malignant tumours

    b. Other unspecified malignant tumours

For this volume, special computer programs were developed in order that the diagnostic data in the NRCT, which are still largely coded according to ICD-O-2 as described earlier, could be mapped onto ICCC-3. This volume contains the first detailed presentation of descriptive epidemiological data on childhood cancer according to ICCC-3 anywhere in the world.

2.6.1 Diagnoses included in the analyses

Throughout this volume, childhood cancer is defined as any diagnosis included in ICCC-3, i.e. all malignant neoplasms together with many non-malignant intracranial and intraspinal tumours. A few diagnoses in groups I and II are excluded, however, mostly because ascertainment is probably very incomplete.

In subgroup Ic (chronic myeloproliferative diseases), polycythaemia vera, chronic myeloproliferative disease, myelosclerosis with myeloid metaplasia and essential thrombocythaemia only received a malignant behaviour code in ICD-O-3. Previously they were regarded as being of uncertain behaviour and were not routinely ascertained by cancer registries. These diseases, all of which are very rare in childhood (McNally et al., 1997), have therefore been excluded from all analyses.

In subgroup Id (myelodysplastic syndrome and other myeloproliferative diseases), the different subtypes of myelodysplastic syndrome (MDS) similarly only acquired a malignant behaviour code in ICD-O-3. They were also excluded from analyses covering periods extending back to before 1991. For 1991–2000, however, they are included, since a high level of ascertainment is believed to have been achieved through the UKCCSG and the UK Paediatric Myelodysplasia Register (Passmore et al., 2003).

In subgroup IId, forms of Langerhans cell histiocytosis (LCH, formerly known as histiocytosis X) with a malignant behaviour code have been excluded. For many years there was doubt as to whether LCH is a true neoplasm, and it was accordingly excluded from ICCC (Kramárová and Stiller 1996). More recently, however, it has been accepted as a clonal disorder and is included in the WHO Classification of Tumours (World Health Organization, 2001) and ICD-O-3. Although the ICD-O-3 classification of LCH includes the terms 'benign' and 'malignant', the more usual distinction among clinicians is between single-system and multi-system disease (Gadner *et al.*, 2001). Historically, few cases of LCH have been registered and coded as such by cancer registries. Although many cases are notified to the NRCT through the UKCCSG, it seems likely that ascertainment is incomplete and virtually certain that the degree of incompleteness has changed over the years.

There is one further modification to the classification as used in this volume, again relating to diagnostic group II. In subgroup IIb, non-Hodgkin lymphoma, division 1, precursor cell lymphomas, includes lymphoblastic lymphoma. While this should be correct for current cases, for most of the period of this study many cases of Burkitt lymphoma, which is in fact a mature B-cell neoplasm, would have been described as lymphoblastic (Wright *et al.*, 1997). Indeed, the Kiel classification, one of the standard classifications for lymphomas, explicitly referred to Burkitt lymphoma as lymphoblastic until it was modified in the late 1980s (Stansfeld *et al.*, 1988). Therefore, cases coded as lymphoblastic lymphoma have only been allocated to the division of precursor cell lymphomas if they were specified as being of T-cell or precursor B-cell lineage; all other cases of lymphoblastic lymphoma have been transferred to subgroup IIb, division 4, non-Hodgkin lymphomas not otherwise specified.

2.7 Geographical coverage and population at risk

The NRCT is a population-based registry which collates all cases of childhood cancer occurring in children normally resident in Great Britain (i.e. England, Wales and Scotland). Northern Ireland is now also included but ascertainment is considered to be complete only from 1993 onwards. Registrations from the Isle of Man are covered by the Merseyside and Cheshire Cancer Registry and should be complete, however numbers are very small and the island is not officially part of Great Britain. The registry also receives notification of some cases occurring among residents of the Channel Islands, but this is probably incomplete. Similarly, some cancers occurring in the children of British armed forces personnel stationed abroad will be notified to the NRCT but are usually excluded from analyses of incidence rates, as are any other children who are normally resident abroad but who come to this country for treatment.

Using postcoded case data together with small area population statistics from annual government publications and the decennial censuses, the CCRG is able to study incidence at various geographical levels. These geographical units range in size from census enumeration districts each containing on average about 85 children, up through wards, county districts, primary care trusts (PCTs), counties, standard regions, countries and finally the whole of Great Britain.

All the analyses of rates and trends presented in this volume are based upon the national data for England, Wales and Scotland only and use mid-year population estimates based on census data together with information on births, deaths and international migration. The estimates are provided by ONS for England and Wales, and GRO for Scotland. Table 2.3 shows the total child population of Great Britain by single year of age in successive decennial censuses from 1971 to 2001.

Table 2.3 Child population of Great Britain by single year of age in selected census years

Age	1971	1981	1991	2001
0	867,303	702,929	767,739	640,827
1	840,261	703,323	749,028	654,660
2	885,084	678,365	744,811	673,868
3	877,328	624,568	756,014	686,912
4	893,330	614,423	734,613	706,194
1–4	**3,496,003**	**2,620,679**	**2,984,466**	**2,721,634**
5	903,971	641,515	727,111	698,888
6	918,413	668,873	723,424	702,003
7	924,317	696,071	694,246	720,005
8	910,252	744,778	697,698	730,693
9	894,634	797,176	697,646	754,824
5–9	**4,551,587**	**3,548,413**	**3,540,125**	**3,606,413**
10	863,387	835,669	708,979	763,949
11	839,123	838,812	713,956	751,593
12	821,831	859,212	687,636	744,693
13	809,123	870,221	634,260	754,881
14	783,670	890,998	624,925	737,207
10–14	**4,117,134**	**4,294,912**	**3,369,756**	**3,752,323**
0–14	**13,032,027**	**11,166,933**	**10,662,086**	**10,721,197**

2.8 Statistical methods

The NRCT data are stored in a SQL Server relational database. For statistical analysis and presentation, data are extracted and exported in suitable formats to various software packages. The statistical analyses presented in this volume were carried out using STATA and Microsoft Excel.

2.8.1 Incidence rates

All incidence rates are expressed as rates per million child years at risk. In the tables, age-specific incidence rates are given for the age groups 0, 1–4, 5–9 and 10–14 years. They are calculated by dividing the number of cases for a specified age–sex group by the corresponding age–sex-specific population at risk. Age-specific rates for single years of age from 0 to 14 were also calculated. Apart from age 0, these do not appear in the tables. They are presented graphically to show the age incidence distributions of the principal diagnostic subgroups and are also used in the calculation of the cumulative rate as described below. Crude incidence rates, calculated by dividing the total number of cases at age 0–14 years by the total child population at risk, are not presented. This is because no cancer has uniform age-specific incidence throughout childhood and therefore the rates would be unduly influenced by variations in the age distribution of the population at risk.

The age-standardized rates (ASRs) are calculated by the direct method using the world standard population, as:

$$\text{ASR} = (2.4r0 + 9.6r1 + 10r2 + 9r3)/31,$$

here $r0$, $r1$, $r2$ and $r3$ are the age-specific rates for age groups 0, 1–4, 5–9 and 10–14 years respectively.

The cumulative rate is the sum of the age-specific incidence rates for single years of age from 0 to 14 and is thus equivalent to 15 times the age-standardized rate calculated with equal weights for the age-specific rates. It is an approximation to the cumulative risk of a child developing the specified cancer in the first 15 years of life in the absence of competing causes of death.

2.8.2 Trends in incidence

Standard Poisson regression methods are used to model annual incidence rates for each diagnostic group, making allowance for the fact that rates differ by age and sex. It is assumed that the incidence rate for each age–sex category is multiplied for each successive year by a factor representing a constant year-on-year change (the trend), which is reported as the average annual percent change (AAPC). The test for trend investigates whether the AAPC, either positive or negative, is significantly different from zero. For some diagnostic groups there is a statistically significant difference between trends in different age groups, or between trends for boys and girls, and, for these, separate AAPCs are reported by age group or sex as appropriate. Ages are grouped in the standard way (0, 1–4, 5–9, 10–14 years old) wherever possible. Adjacent age groups are combined if this is necessary to achieve at least one case in each age–sex category: Hodgkin lymphoma, osteosarcoma, female gonadal germ cell tumours, thyroid and other/unspecified carcinomas (0–4, 5–9, 10–14); unilateral retinoblastoma (0, 1–4, 5–14); bilateral retinoblastoma (0, 1–14). For some diagnostic groups (marked in the tables of results) there is evidence of lack of fit to the model, from the deviance goodness-of-fit statistic. In these groups, the AAPC is probably valid as an average rate of change, but the confidence intervals and trend test results may be inaccurate.

2.8.3 Survival analysis

Actuarial survival curves are constructed from the Kaplan–Meier product-limit estimate of the survivor function. Log-rank tests are used to test the equality of survivor functions across one or more groups and to test for time trends in survival (Peto *et al.*, 1977).

2.8.4 Mortality

For the analyses of mortality, the cases are classified wherever possible according to the diagnosis recorded at the time of the initial presentation and not according to the specified cause of death. However, if no other information is available then the malignancy recorded on the death certificate is used. Hence all children diagnosed with cancer who died before the age of 15 years from whatever cause (whether related to the malignancy or not) are included in this analysis. The age and dates referred to are those at the time of the death of the child and may well be different to those at the time of initial diagnosis.

Data are presented for the whole of England, Wales and Scotland for the age-groups 0, 1–4, 5–9 and 10–14. For the twelve main diagnostic groups and for all cancers, combined analyses are given in five-year calendar periods from 1965 to 2004. Data are also presented for the main diagnostic groups, and selected sub-groups, for the most recent ten-year period available, 1995–2004.

In addition to the presentation of numbers and age-specific rates, the tables also give the ASR calculated in the same way as for the incidence tables using the world standard population.

Also presented is an illustration of the percentage of all deaths in childhood which occur among children diagnosed with a malignant neoplasm (or non-malignant brain tumour). The denominator used here is the published ONS data by age-group for deaths from all causes.

Chapter 3

Incidence of Childhood Cancer 1991–2000

CA Stiller, ME Kroll and EM Eatock

In this chapter, we describe in detail the incidence of childhood cancer in Great Britain during the decade 1991–2000. Incidence rates are presented by age and sex for all cancers combined and for the diagnostic groups, subgroups and divisions of ICCC-3. Additional information is given on immunophenotype for lymphoid neoplasms, French–American–British (FAB) classification for acute myeloid leukaemia (AML), histological subtype for selected subgroups or divisions, primary site for solid tumours, and laterality for retinoblastoma and nephroblastoma (Wilms tumour). Most of the results are presented in tables, but incidence rates by single year of age are shown graphically for the principal diagnostic categories.

The results are discussed in relation to those from other studies. The variations in childhood cancer occurrence between different world regions are well documented (Parkin et al., 1988a, 1998; Stiller and Parkin, 1996). Here, we concentrate on comparisons with population-based studies in other industrialized countries with mainly white Caucasian populations in Europe, North America and Oceania. The largest relevant studies are International Incidence of Childhood Cancer, Volume 2 (IICC-2) (Parkin et al., 1998) for all regions of the world, the Automated Childhood Cancer Information System (ACCIS) (Steliarova-Foucher et al., 2004, 2006a) for Europe, and the Surveillance, Epidemiology and End Results (SEER) Program Pediatric Cancer Monograph (Ries et al., 1999) for the United States. The data in IICC-2 mostly cover the 1980s and the SEER study goes up to 1995. The ACCIS study goes up to 1997 but the results are generally presented by European region rather than for individual countries. In the more detailed presentation of the ACCIS data, however, one of the five regions is the British Isles, consisting of the UK and Ireland (Steliarova-Foucher et al., 2006a). Data from the 1990s have been published from several individual countries. In France, incidence data have been published from the National Registry of Childhood Leukaemia and Lymphoma (Clavel et al., 2004) and, for solid tumours, from the pooled data of six regional or departmental childhood cancer registries covering 32% of the child population (Desandes et al., 2004). The German Childhood Cancer Registry (2002) has published incidence rates in its annual reports and detailed results on CNS tumours (Kaatsch et al., 2001). Incidence data for the Netherlands have been published by the Netherlands Cancer Registry (2000). A report on secular trends in childhood cancer incidence in Sweden (Dreifaldt et al., 2004) included incidence rates for 1990–98. Incidence data from

New Zealand have been published for 1990–93 based on the results of a pathology review (Dockerty *et al.*, 1997; Becroft *et al.*, 1999).

While all the paediatric cancer registries and some European general cancer registries include non-malignant CNS tumours, the SEER registries for the period covered by the *Pediatric Cancer Monograph* restricted their coverage to malignant neoplasms. The Central Brain Tumor Registry of the United States (CBTRUS), however, includes non-malignant tumours and has published incidence data for 1995–99 (CBTRUS, 2002).

The studies mentioned above have all classified diagnoses according to the International Classification of Childhood Cancer (Kramárovà and Stiller, 1996) or, in the case of those devoted to haematological neoplasms or CNS tumours, have used more detailed classification schemes.

The discussion in this chapter refers to population-based studies where possible, but for some points there are few or no population data available and we have then had recourse to clinical studies.

3.1 Total incidence

During the ten-year study period, there was a total of 14,659 registrations for all types of childhood cancer. This figure excludes 118 cases of second malignant neoplasms diagnosed in childhood during this period. Table 3.1 shows the numbers of registrations by age and sex for all cancers combined and for the diagnostic groups and subgroups of ICCC-3. Table 3.2 shows incidence rates based on the same data. The total age-standardized annual incidence rate was 139 per million children aged under 15 years. The cumulative incidence was 2027 per million, which is equivalent to a risk of 1 in 493 of developing cancer in the first 15 years of life. Incidence was highest, 188 per million, among infants aged under a year and slightly less, 186 per million, among children aged 1–4 years. Incidence rates at ages 5–9 and 10–14 years were considerably lower, 108 and 111 per million respectively. Figure 3.1 shows incidence rates by single year of age for boys and girls. Cancer was more common among boys than girls throughout childhood. The male excess was proportionally somewhat higher at age 5–9 years than in the other age groups.

Overall, the most frequent diagnostic groups were leukaemias, CNS tumours, lymphomas, neuroblastoma and other peripheral nervous cell tumours, soft tissue sarcomas and renal tumours, each of which accounted for between 33 and 6% of the total age-standardized incidence (Fig. 3.2). The contributions of the main diagnostic groups varied markedly with age and between the sexes (Figs. 3.3–3.8). Leukaemias formed the most common group overall, and their incidence was more than twice that of the next most frequent group at age 1–4 years. They were the most frequent group among infants by a much smaller margin, however, and were outnumbered by CNS tumours at ages 5–9 and 10–14 years. Leukaemias and CNS tumours had the highest and second highest incidence respectively among both boys and girls. Lymphomas were the third most frequent group overall and among boys, but soft tissue sarcomas ranked third among girls.

The total incidence of childhood cancer was at the lower end of the range observed in western industrialized countries (Parkin *et al.*, 1998; Ries *et al.*, 1999; Stiller *et al.*, 2006b).

Text starts on page 38

Table 3.1 Numbers of registrations for childhood cancer, including non-malignant CNS tumours, Great Britain, 1991–2000

| | Registrations for age group (years) at diagnosis | | | | | | | | | | | | | | | |
| | Boys | | | | | Girls | | | | | Children | | | | | |
	0	1–4	5–9	10–14	Total	0	1–4	5–9	10–14	Total	0	1–4	5–9	10–14	Total	MV
Leukaemias, myeloproliferative and myelodysplastic diseases	**143**	**1263**	**740**	**505**	**2651**	**130**	**1016**	**526**	**372**	**2044**	**273**	**2279**	**1266**	**879**	**4695**	**0.98**
Lymphoid leukaemias	62	1087	609	349	2107	66	857	432	253	1608	128	1944	1041	602	3715	0.99
Acute myeloid leukaemias	54	117	94	119	384	42	114	67	86	309	96	231	161	205	693	0.97
Chronic myeloproliferative diseases	0	4	10	22	36	0	4	8	15	27	0	8	18	37	63	0.92
Myelodysplastic syndrome and other myeloproliferative diseases	20	47	24	8	99	15	32	13	14	74	35	79	37	22	173	0.96
Unspecified and other specified leukaemias	7	8	3	7	25	7	9	6	4	26	14	17	9	11	51	0.67
Lymphomas and reticuloendothelial neoplasms	**5**	**164**	**346**	**471**	**986**	**3**	**67**	**128**	**240**	**438**	**8**	**231**	**474**	**711**	**1424**	**0.96**
Hodgkin lymphomas	0	31	107	247	385	0	8	46	145	199	0	39	153	392	584	0.97
Non-Hodgkin lymphomas (except Burkitt lymphoma)	4	90	170	168	432	2	49	61	80	192	6	139	231	248	624	0.96
Burkitt lymphoma	0	39	64	47	150	0	8	18	15	41	0	47	82	62	191	1.00
Miscellaneous lymphoreticular neoplasms	1	2	0	2	5	1	1	1	0	3	2	3	1	2	8	0.75
Unspecified lymphomas	0	2	5	7	14	0	1	2	0	3	0	3	7	7	17	0.41
CNS and miscellaneous intracranial and intraspinal neoplasms	**136**	**559**	**686**	**525**	**1906**	**115**	**491**	**616**	**477**	**1699**	**251**	**1050**	**1302**	**1002**	**3605**	**0.79**

Table 3.1 (continued) Numbers of registrations for childhood cancer, including non-malignant CNS tumours, Great Britain, 1991–2000

	Registrations for age group (years) at diagnosis															
	Boys					Girls					Children					
	0	1–4	5–9	10–14	Total	0	1–4	5–9	10–14	Total	0	1–4	5–9	10–14	Total	MV
Ependymomas and choroid plexus tumour	28	104	49	27	208	21	57	33	33	144	49	161	82	60	352	0.95
Astrocytomas	40	199	278	222	739	34	240	301	237	812	74	439	579	459	1551	0.85
Intracranial and intraspinal embryonal tumours	35	136	161	91	423	29	99	105	41	274	64	235	266	132	697	0.97
Other gliomas	8	50	86	48	192	6	43	80	59	188	14	93	166	107	380	0.28
Other specified intracranial and intraspinal neoplasms	13	47	91	102	253	15	34	67	83	199	28	81	158	185	452	0.85
Unspecified intracranial and intraspinal neoplasms	12	23	21	35	91	10	18	30	24	82	22	41	51	59	173	0.15
Neuroblastoma and other peripheral nervous cell tumours	**142**	**290**	**62**	**11**	**505**	**115**	**219**	**48**	**10**	**392**	**257**	**509**	**110**	**21**	**897**	**0.97**
Neuroblastoma and ganglioneuroblastoma	142	287	60	10	499	115	218	46	8	387	257	505	106	18	886	0.97
Other peripheral nervous cell tumours	0	3	2	1	6	0	1	2	2	5	0	4	4	3	11	1.00
Retinoblastoma	**99**	**107**	**10**	**2**	**218**	**82**	**122**	**8**	**0**	**212**	**181**	**229**	**18**	**2**	**430**	**0.73**
Renal tumours	**63**	**253**	**78**	**20**	**414**	**50**	**255**	**67**	**25**	**397**	**113**	**508**	**145**	**45**	**811**	**0.97**
Nephroblastoma and other nonepithelial renal tumours	61	251	74	14	400	50	255	65	17	387	111	506	139	31	787	0.98
Renal carcinomas	0	2	2	6	10	0	0	1	8	9	0	2	3	14	19	1.00
Unspecified malignant renal tumours	2	0	2	0	4	0	0	1	0	1	2	0	3	0	5	0.20

Hepatic tumours	24	43	7	10	84	18	21	5	10	54	42	64	12	20	**138**	**0.95**
Hepatoblastoma	24	39	4	4	71	18	21	1	1	41	42	60	5	5	112	0.96
Hepatic carcinomas	0	3	3	6	12	0	0	4	9	13	0	3	7	15	25	0.96
Unspecified malignant hepatic tumours	0	1	0	0	1	0	0	0	0	0	0	1	0	0	1	0.00
Malignant bone tumours	1	11	73	199	284	4	14	77	184	279	5	25	150	383	**563**	**0.96**
Osteosarcomas	0	1	42	105	148	0	4	46	109	159	0	5	88	214	307	0.98
Chondrosarcomas	0	0	0	9	9	1	0	0	2	3	1	0	0	11	12	0.75
Ewing tumour and related bone sarcomas	0	9	30	78	117	1	10	27	62	100	1	19	57	140	217	0.99
Other specified malignant bone tumours	0	0	0	6	6	1	0	2	7	10	1	0	2	13	16	1.00
Unspecified malignant bone tumours	1	1	1	1	4	1	0	2	4	7	2	1	3	5	11	0.36
Soft tissue and other extraosseous sarcomas	56	190	172	156	574	49	133	125	147	454	105	323	297	303	**1028**	**0.96**
Rhabdomyosarcomas	26	151	107	46	330	21	97	63	36	217	47	248	170	82	547	0.98
Fibrosarcomas, peripheral nerve sheath tumours and other fibrous neoplasms	9	4	8	13	34	7	5	10	24	46	16	9	18	37	80	0.94
Kaposi sarcoma	0	0	1	1	2	0	0	2	1	3	0	0	3	2	5	0.40
Other specified soft tissue sarcomas	17	30	51	81	179	15	28	40	78	161	32	58	91	159	340	0.94
Unspecified soft tissue sarcomas	4	5	5	15	29	6	3	10	8	27	10	8	15	23	56	0.96
Germ cell tumours, trophoblastic tumours and neoplasms of gonads	48	65	27	88	228	32	58	54	114	258	80	123	81	202	**486**	**0.92**
Intracranial and intraspinal germ cell tumours	8	5	25	61	99	6	13	17	30	66	14	18	42	91	165	0.84

Table 3.1 (continued) Numbers of registrations for childhood cancer, including non-malignant CNS tumours, Great Britain, 1991–2000

| | Registrations for age group (years) at diagnosis | | | | | | | | | | | | | | | |
| | Boys | | | | | Girls | | | | | Children | | | | | |
	0	1–4	5–9	10–14	Total	0	1–4	5–9	10–14	Total	0	1–4	5–9	10–14	Total	MV
Malignant extracranial and extragonadal germ cell tumours	17	13	1	3	34	26	39	3	5	73	43	52	4	8	107	0.95
Malignant gonadal germ cell tumours	22	47	1	22	92	0	6	31	75	112	22	53	32	97	204	0.97
Gonadal carcinomas	0	0	0	1	1	0	0	3	4	7	0	0	3	5	8	0.88
Other and unspecified malignant gonadal tumours	1	0	0	1	2	0	0	0	0	0	1	0	0	1	2	0.00
Other malignant epithelial neoplasms and malignant melanomas	4	16	44	155	219	6	30	61	167	264	10	46	105	322	483	0.83
Adrenocortical carcinomas	1	6	0	0	7	1	7	5	4	17	2	13	5	4	24	1.00
Thyroid carcinomas	0	3	6	16	25	0	2	11	33	46	0	5	17	49	71	0.93
Nasopharyngeal carcinomas	0	0	3	17	20	0	0	0	4	4	0	0	3	21	24	0.96
Malignant melanomas	2	3	17	43	65	5	16	22	46	89	7	19	39	89	154	0.80
Skin carcinomas	1	2	10	31	44	0	3	10	25	38	1	5	20	56	82	0.71
Other and unspecified carcinomas	0	2	8	48	58	0	2	13	55	70	0	4	21	103	128	0.77
Other and unspecified malignant neoplasms	8	10	12	14	44	7	22	8	18	55	15	32	20	32	99	0.22
Other specified malignant tumours	1	3	1	3	8	1	5	0	3	9	2	8	1	6	17	1.00
Other unspecified malignant tumours	7	7	11	11	36	6	17	8	15	46	13	24	19	26	82	0.06
Total	729	2971	2257	2156	8113	611	2448	1723	1764	6546	1340	5419	3980	3920	14,659	0.91

MV, proportion of cases with microscopic verification

Table 3.2 Annual age-specific and age-standardized incidence rates for childhood cancer, including non-malignant CNS tumours, Great Britain, 1991–2000

| | Annual incidence per million children for age group (years) at diagnosis | | | | | | | | | | | | | | | | |
| | Boys | | | | | Girls | | | | | Children | | | | | |
	0	1–4	5–9	10–14	Total ASR	0	1–4	5–9	10–14	Total ASR	0	1–4	5–9	10–14	Total ASR	M/F
Leukaemias, myeloproliferative and myelodysplastic diseases	**39.15**	**84.65**	**39.36**	**27.93**	**50.05**	**37.38**	**71.37**	**29.28**	**21.49**	**40.68**	**38.28**	**78.17**	**34.44**	**24.78**	**45.47**	**1.23**
Lymphoid leukaemias	16.97	72.85	32.39	19.30	39.93	18.98	60.20	24.05	14.62	32.11	17.95	66.68	28.32	17.01	36.11	1.24
Acute myeloid leukaemias	14.78	7.84	5.00	6.58	7.10	12.08	8.01	3.73	4.97	6.06	13.46	7.92	4.38	5.79	6.59	1.17
Chronic myeloproliferative diseases	0.00	0.27	0.53	1.22	0.61	0.00	0.28	0.45	0.87	0.48	0.00	0.27	0.49	1.05	0.55	1.26
Myelodysplastic syndrome and other myeloproliferative diseases	5.48	3.15	1.28	0.44	1.94	4.31	2.25	0.72	0.81	1.50	4.91	2.71	1.01	0.62	1.72	1.29
Unspecified and other specified leukaemias	1.92	0.54	0.16	0.39	0.48	2.01	0.63	0.33	0.23	0.53	1.96	0.58	0.24	0.31	0.50	0.91
Lymphomas and reticuloendothelial neoplasms	**1.37**	**10.99**	**18.40**	**26.05**	**17.01**	**0.86**	**4.71**	**7.13**	**13.86**	**7.85**	**1.12**	**7.92**	**12.89**	**20.09**	**12.53**	**2.17**
Hodgkin lymphomas	0.00	2.08	5.69	13.66	6.45	0.00	0.56	2.56	8.38	3.43	0.00	1.34	4.16	11.08	4.97	1.88
Non-Hodgkin lymphomas (except Burkitt lymphoma)	1.10	6.03	9.04	9.29	7.57	0.58	3.44	3.40	4.62	3.55	0.84	4.77	6.28	7.01	5.60	2.13
Burkitt lymphoma	0.00	2.61	3.40	2.60	2.66	0.00	0.56	1.00	0.87	0.75	0.00	1.61	2.23	1.75	1.73	3.56
Miscellaneous lymphoreticular neoplasms	0.27	0.13	0.00	0.11	0.09	0.29	0.07	0.06	0.00	0.06	0.28	0.10	0.03	0.06	0.08	1.53
Unspecified lymphomas	0.00	0.13	0.27	0.39	0.24	0.00	0.07	0.11	0.00	0.06	0.00	0.10	0.19	0.20	0.15	4.16

Table 3.2 (continued) Annual age-specific and age-standardized incidence rates for childhood cancer, including non-malignant CNS tumours, Great Britain, 1991–2000

	Annual incidence per million children for age group (years) at diagnosis															
	Boys					Girls					Children					
	0	1–4	5–9	10–14	Total ASR	0	1–4	5–9	10–14	Total ASR	0	1–4	5–9	10–14	Total ASR	M/F
CNS and miscellaneous intracranial and intraspinal neoplasms	37.23	37.46	36.49	29.04	34.69	33.06	34.49	34.29	27.56	32.30	35.20	36.01	35.42	28.31	33.52	1.07
Ependymomas and choroid plexus tumour	7.67	6.97	2.61	1.49	4.03	6.04	4.00	1.84	1.91	2.85	6.87	5.52	2.23	1.70	3.45	1.41
Astrocytomas	10.95	13.34	14.79	12.28	13.31	9.78	16.86	16.76	13.69	15.36	10.38	15.06	15.75	12.97	14.31	0.87
Intracranial and intraspinal embryonal tumours	9.58	9.11	8.56	5.03	7.79	8.34	6.95	5.85	2.37	5.37	8.97	8.06	7.24	3.73	6.61	1.45
Other gliomas	2.19	3.35	4.57	2.66	3.45	1.73	3.02	4.45	3.41	3.50	1.96	3.19	4.52	3.02	3.47	0.99
Other specified intracranial and intraspinal neoplasms	3.56	3.15	4.84	5.64	4.45	4.31	2.39	3.73	4.79	3.67	3.93	2.78	4.30	5.23	4.07	1.21
Unspecified intracranial and intraspinal neoplasms	3.29	1.54	1.12	1.94	1.65	2.88	1.26	1.67	1.39	1.56	3.09	1.41	1.39	1.67	1.61	1.06
Neuroblastoma and other peripheral nervous cell tumours	38.87	19.44	3.30	0.61	10.27	33.06	15.38	2.67	0.58	8.35	36.04	17.46	2.99	0.59	9.33	1.23
Neuroblastoma and ganglioneuroblastoma	38.87	19.23	3.19	0.55	10.16	33.06	15.31	2.56	0.46	8.26	36.04	17.32	2.88	0.51	9.23	1.23
Other peripheral nervous cell tumours	0.00	0.20	0.11	0.06	0.11	0.00	0.07	0.11	0.12	0.09	0.00	0.14	0.11	0.08	0.10	1.23
Retinoblastoma	27.10	7.17	0.53	0.11	4.52	23.58	8.57	0.45	0.00	4.62	25.38	7.85	0.49	0.06	4.57	0.98
Renal tumours	17.25	16.96	4.15	1.11	8.25	14.38	17.91	3.73	1.44	8.28	15.85	17.42	3.94	1.27	8.26	1.00

Nephroblastoma and other nonepithelial renal tumours	16.70	16.82	3.94	0.77	8.00	14.38	17.91	3.62	0.98	8.11	15.57	17.35	3.78	0.88	8.05	0.99
Renal carcinomas	0.00	0.13	0.11	0.33	0.17	0.00	0.00	0.06	0.46	0.15	0.00	0.07	0.08	0.40	0.16	1.13
Unspecified malignant renal tumours	0.55	0.00	0.11	0.00	0.08	0.00	0.00	0.06	0.00	0.02	0.28	0.00	0.08	0.00	0.05	4.27
Hepatic tumours	**6.57**	**2.88**	**0.37**	**0.55**	**1.68**	**5.18**	**1.48**	**0.28**	**0.58**	**1.12**	**5.89**	**2.20**	**0.33**	**0.57**	**1.41**	**1.51**
Hepatoblastoma	6.57	2.61	0.21	0.22	1.45	5.18	1.48	0.06	0.06	0.89	5.89	2.06	0.14	0.14	1.18	1.63
Hepatic carcinomas	0.00	0.20	0.16	0.33	0.21	0.00	0.00	0.22	0.52	0.22	0.00	0.10	0.19	0.42	0.22	0.94
Unspecified malignant hepatic tumours	0.00	0.07	0.00	0.00	0.02	0.00	0.00	0.00	0.00	0.00	0.00	0.03	0.00	0.00	0.01	–
Malignant bone tumours	**0.27**	**0.74**	**3.88**	**11.01**	**4.70**	**1.15**	**0.98**	**4.29**	**10.63**	**4.86**	**0.70**	**0.86**	**4.08**	**10.82**	**4.78**	**0.97**
Osteosarcomas	0.00	0.07	2.23	5.81	2.43	0.00	0.28	2.56	6.30	2.74	0.00	0.17	2.39	6.05	2.58	0.89
Chondrosarcomas	0.00	0.00	0.00	0.50	0.14	0.29	0.00	0.00	0.12	0.06	0.14	0.00	0.00	0.31	0.10	2.59
Ewing tumour and related bone sarcomas	0.00	0.60	1.60	4.31	1.95	0.29	0.70	1.50	3.58	1.76	0.14	0.65	1.55	3.96	1.86	1.11
Other specified malignant bone tumours	0.00	0.00	0.00	0.33	0.10	0.29	0.00	0.11	0.40	0.18	0.14	0.00	0.05	0.37	0.14	0.55
Unspecified malignant bone tumours	0.27	0.07	0.05	0.06	0.08	0.29	0.00	0.11	0.23	0.13	0.28	0.03	0.08	0.14	0.10	0.60
Soft tissue and other extraosseous sarcomas	**15.33**	**12.73**	**9.15**	**8.62**	**10.59**	**14.09**	**9.34**	**6.96**	**8.49**	**8.69**	**14.72**	**11.08**	**8.08**	**8.56**	**9.66**	**1.22**
Rhabdomyosarcomas	7.12	10.12	5.69	2.54	6.26	6.04	6.81	3.51	2.08	4.31	6.59	8.51	4.62	2.32	5.31	1.45
Fibrosarcomas, peripheral nerve sheath tumours and other fibrous neoplasms	2.46	0.27	0.43	0.72	0.62	2.01	0.35	0.56	1.39	0.85	2.24	0.31	0.49	1.05	0.73	0.73
Kaposi sarcoma	0.00	0.00	0.05	0.06	0.03	0.00	0.00	0.11	0.06	0.05	0.00	0.00	0.08	0.06	0.04	0.63

Table 3.2 (continued) Annual age-specific and age-standardized incidence rates for childhood cancer, including non-malignant CNS tumours, Great Britain, 1991–2000

Annual incidence per million children for age group (years) at diagnosis

	Boys					Girls					Children					
	0	1–4	5–9	10–14	Total ASR	0	1–4	5–9	10–14	Total ASR	0	1–4	5–9	10–14	Total ASR	M/F
Other specified soft tissue sarcomas	4.65	2.01	2.71	4.48	3.16	4.31	1.97	2.23	4.51	2.97	4.49	1.99	2.48	4.49	3.07	1.06
Unspecified soft tissue sarcomas	1.10	0.34	0.27	0.83	0.52	1.73	0.21	0.56	0.46	0.51	1.40	0.27	0.41	0.65	0.51	1.01
Germ cell tumours, trophoblastic tumours and neoplasms of gonads	**13.14**	**4.36**	**1.44**	**4.87**	**4.24**	**9.20**	**4.07**	**3.01**	**6.59**	**4.86**	**11.22**	**4.22**	**2.20**	**5.71**	**4.54**	**0.87**
Intracranial and intraspinal germ cell tumours	2.19	0.34	1.33	3.37	1.68	1.73	0.91	0.95	1.73	1.22	1.96	0.62	1.14	2.57	1.46	1.37
Malignant extracranial and extragonadal germ cell tumours	4.65	0.87	0.05	0.17	0.70	7.48	2.74	0.17	0.29	1.56	6.03	1.78	0.11	0.23	1.12	0.44
Malignant gonadal germ cell tumours	6.02	3.15	0.05	1.22	1.81	0.00	0.42	1.73	4.33	1.95	3.09	1.82	0.87	2.74	1.88	0.93
Gonadal carcinomas	0.00	0.00	0.00	0.06	0.02	0.00	0.00	0.17	0.23	0.12	0.00	0.00	0.08	0.14	0.07	0.13
Other and unspecified malignant gonadal tumours	0.27	0.00	0.00	0.06	0.04	0.00	0.00	0.00	0.00	0.00	0.14	0.00	0.00	0.03	0.02	–
Other malignant epithelial neoplasms and malignant melanomas	**1.10**	**1.07**	**2.34**	**8.57**	**3.66**	**1.73**	**2.11**	**3.40**	**9.64**	**4.68**	**1.40**	**1.58**	**2.86**	**9.10**	**4.16**	**0.78**
Adrenocortical carcinomas	0.27	0.40	0.00	0.00	0.15	0.29	0.49	0.28	0.23	0.33	0.28	0.45	0.14	0.11	0.24	0.44
Thyroid carcinomas	0.00	0.20	0.32	0.89	0.42	0.00	0.14	0.61	1.91	0.79	0.00	0.17	0.46	1.38	0.60	0.53

Nasopharyngeal carcinomas		0.00	0.00	0.16	0.94	0.32	0.00	0.00	0.23	0.07	0.00	0.00	0.08	0.59	0.20	4.84
Malignant melanomas		0.55	0.20	0.90	2.38	1.09	1.12	1.22	2.66	1.63	0.98	0.65	1.06	2.51	1.35	0.67
Skin carcinomas		0.27	0.13	0.53	1.71	0.73	0.21	0.56	1.44	0.66	0.14	0.17	0.54	1.58	0.70	1.10
Other and unspecified carcinomas		0.00	0.13	0.43	2.66	0.95	0.14	0.72	3.18	1.20	0.00	0.14	0.57	2.91	1.07	0.79
Other and unspecified malignant neoplasms		**2.19**	**0.67**	**0.64**	**0.77**	**0.81**	**1.55**	**0.45**	**1.04**	**1.08**	**2.10**	**1.10**	**0.54**	**0.90**	**0.94**	**0.75**
Other specified malignant tumours		0.27	0.20	0.05	0.17	0.15	0.35	0.00	0.17	0.18	0.28	0.27	0.03	0.17	0.16	0.82
Other unspecified malignant tumours		1.92	0.47	0.59	0.61	0.66	1.19	0.45	0.87	0.90	1.82	0.82	0.52	0.73	0.78	0.73
Total	199.57	199.11	120.05	119.25	150.46	175.67	171.97	95.92	101.91	127.38	187.91	185.86	108.26	110.77	139.19	1.18

ASR, age-standardized rate based on World Standard Population

M/F, ratio of ASR for boys to ASR for girls

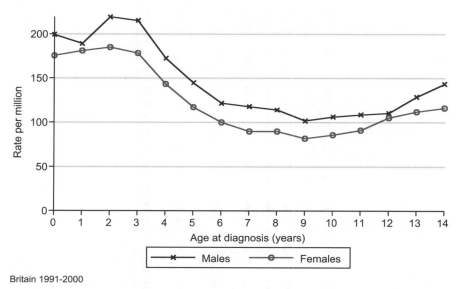

Britain 1991-2000

Fig. 3.1 Annual incidence rates by single year of age for all childhood cancers by sex, Great Britain, 1991–2000.

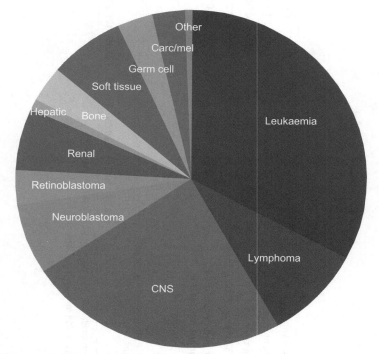

Fig. 3.2 Relative contributions of the 12 diagnostic groups of childhood cancer to age-standardized incidence among children aged 0–14 years, Great Britain, 1991–2000.

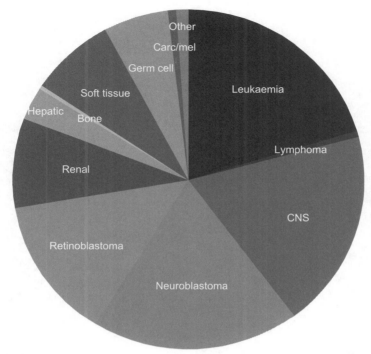

Fig. 3.3 Relative contributions of the 12 diagnostic groups of childhood cancer to incidence among infants aged under 1 year, Great Britain, 1991–2000.

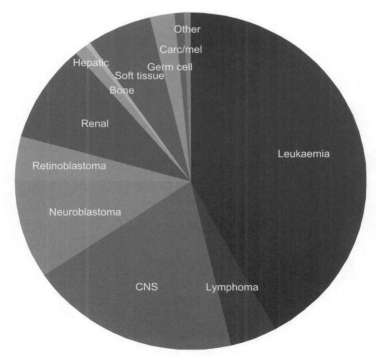

Fig. 3.4 Relative contributions of the 12 diagnostic groups of childhood cancer to incidence among children aged 1–4 years, Great Britain, 1991–2000.

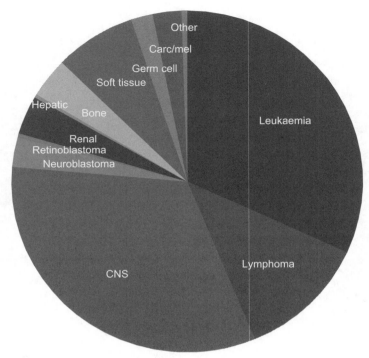

Fig. 3.5 Relative contributions of the 12 diagnostic groups of childhood cancer to incidence among children aged 5–9 years, Great Britain, 1991–2000.

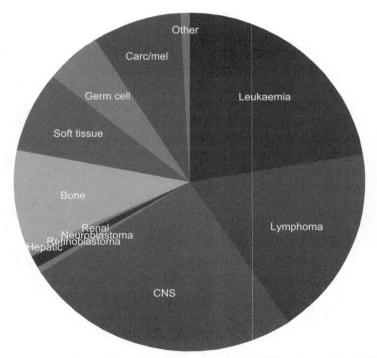

Fig. 3.6 Relative contributions of the 12 diagnostic groups of childhood cancer to incidence among children aged 10–14 years, Great Britain, 1991–2000.

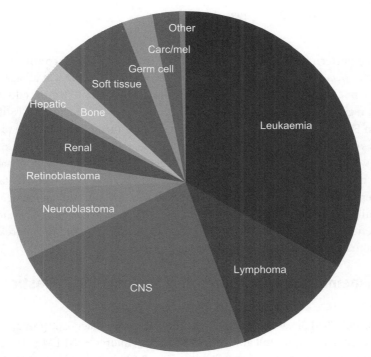

Fig. 3.7 Relative contributions of the 12 diagnostic groups of childhood cancer to age-standardized incidence among boys aged 0–14 years, Great Britain, 1991–2000.

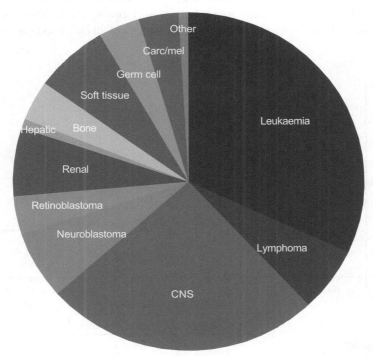

Fig. 3.8 Relative contributions of the 12 diagnostic groups of childhood cancer to age-standardized incidence among girls aged 0–14 years, Great Britain, 1991–2000.

The overall pattern was broadly similar to that in other western countries, with the highest rates occurring in the first 5 years of life, an excess of boys at all ages, and the predominance of leukaemias and CNS tumours. The deficit compared with other European regions was, however, particularly pronounced among infants (Stiller *et al.*, 2006b). In France, for example, total cancer incidence throughout the age range 1–14 years was very similar to that in Britain, but infants had an incidence rate of 223 per million, 19% greater than in Britain (Desandes *et al.*, 2004); this was entirely accounted for by the much higher incidence of neuroblastoma in France. In the United States, there was an even larger excess among infants compared with Britain, with an incidence rate of 269 per million during 1986–94 despite the fact that non-malignant CNS neoplasms were excluded (Gurney *et al.*, 1999b). The excess was most marked for neuroblastoma, renal tumours, hepatic tumours and germ cell tumours.

3.2 Leukaemias, myeloproliferative and myelodysplastic diseases

Leukaemia and allied diseases constituted the most common diagnostic group, accounting for 32% of registrations overall and 42% of those for children aged 1–4 years. There was a marked peak in incidence at age 2–3 years (Fig. 3.9). Leukaemia was more frequent among boys than girls at all ages, but the difference was very small in the first year of life. Lymphoid leukaemia, which in childhood is equivalent to acute lymphoblastic leukaemia (ALL), was the largest diagnostic subgroup not only among the leukaemias but also among childhood cancer as a whole. It accounted for 25% of all childhood cancers and for

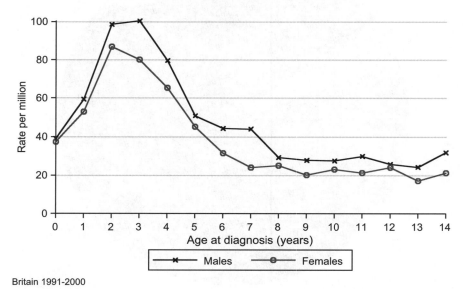

Britain 1991-2000

Fig. 3.9 Annual incidence rates by single year of age for leukaemias, myeloproliferative and myelodysplastic diseases, by sex, Great Britain, 1991–2000.

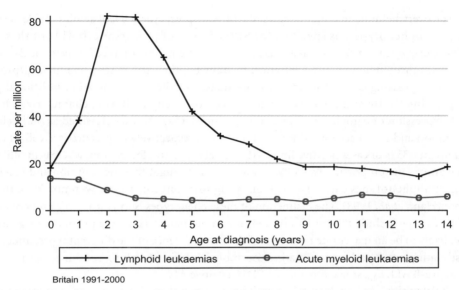

Britain 1991-2000

Fig. 3.10 Annual incidence rates by single year of age for lymphoid leukaemias and acute myeloid leukaemias, Great Britain, 1991–2000.

36% of those at age 1–4 years; 79% of leukaemias were ALL. The highest incidence was at age 2–3 years (Fig. 3.10). The peak was at age 2 years for girls but 3 years for boys (Fig. 3.11). Overall there was a male excess, with a male:female ratio of ASRs of 1.24:1. The male excess was slightly more marked at age 5–14, in excess of 1.3:1; among infants aged under 1 year, there was a higher incidence rate for females, and the sex ratio was 0.89:1.

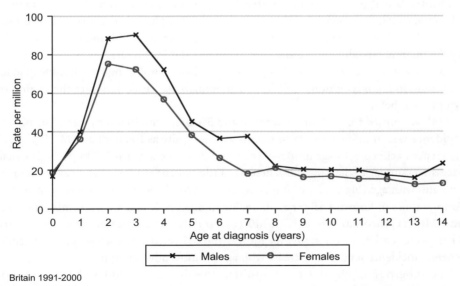

Britain 1991-2000

Fig. 3.11 Annual incidence rates by single year of age for lymphoid leukaemias, by sex, Great Britain, 1991–2000.

The overwhelming majority of cases of ALL were precursor cell leukaemias (Table 3.3). Immunophenotype was specified for 81% of cases of precursor cell ALL; of these, 87% were precursor B-cell leukaemias and 13% were precursor T-cell. Precursor B-cell ALL has three stages of differentiation recognized: the earliest stage is null-cell/pre-pre-B, expressing CD19; the intermediate stage, so-called common ALL, additionally expressing CD10; and the most mature stage, so-called pre-B ALL, characterized by the expression of cytoplasmic mu chains (cyt-mu). Overall cases classified as null-cell, common and pre-B accounted for 5, 81 and 14%, respectively of precursor B-cell ALL. In infants, 33% of cases positive for CD10 were also positive for cyt-mu, whereas in other age groups the proportion was 14%. It was initially thought that the common and pre-B immunophenotypes carried a different prognosis but this has proven not to be the case (Hann et al., 1998). The distinction of these phenotypes is thus academic and not all centres now include the cyt-mu in their screening panel. Thus, the proportions given are likely to be an inaccurate reflection of the true incidence of the different types, under-estimating pre-B and overestimating common. We have, therefore, combined common and pre-B ALL in a single category of CD10 positive ALL.

CD10 positive ALL had a marked peak in incidence at age 1–4 years and accounted for 91% of cases of known subtype in this age group. It was rare in infants aged under a year. Null-cell ALL had its highest incidence in infancy; 41% of cases were in children aged under a year and within this age group null-cell ALL accounted for 58% of cases of known subtype. T-cell ALL was very rare in the first year of life and there was a moderate peak at age 5–9 years. The sex ratio also varied between immunophenotypes. For CD10 positive ALL the male:female ratio was 1.21:1. The male excess was more marked for T-cell ALL, 1.84:1, and relatively small for null-cell ALL, 1.08:1.

Mature B-cell leukaemia accounted for 1.5% of cases of lymphoid leukaemia. All of these cases were B-cell ALL; no cases of chronic lymphatic leukaemia were registered. Mature T-cell or NK-cell leukaemia has been recorded in childhood (Gardiner et al., 1995), but it is exceedingly rare and there were no cases in this series.

Patterns of total incidence for lymphoid neoplasms, combining lymphoid leukaemia and non-Hodgkin lymphoma (NHL), are presented and discussed after the section on lymphomas below.

AML accounted for 15% of leukaemias and 5% of all childhood cancers. The highest incidence was in infants, but even then it was not quite as frequent as ALL (Fig. 3.12). Incidence declined with age until 5–9 years and then rose again at 10–14 years. The male excess was similar to that for ALL. There was little evidence of systematic variation in the sex ratio with age (Fig. 3.12). FAB type was known for 74% of cases of AML (Table 3.4). Among those of known FAB type, M5 (acute monocytic leukaemia) was most frequent, and M6 (erythroleukaemia) and M0 (minimally differentiated) were very rare. There were marked peaks in infancy for M5 and M7 (acute megakaryocytic leukaemia) whereas incidence tended to increase with age for most other subtypes.

The subgroup of chronic myeloproliferative diseases includes chronic myeloid leukaemia (CML) together with chronic neutrophilic and eosinophilic leukaemia, polycythaemia vera, myelosclerosis with myeloid metaplasia, essential thrombocythaemia

Table 3.3 Numbers of registrations and age-standardized annual incidence per million children for lymphoid leukaemias by immunophenotype, Great Britain, 1991–2000

Age group (years) at diagnosis	Registrations				Total			ASR		
Children	**0**	**1–4**	**5–9**	**10–14**	**Boys**	**Girls**	**Children**	**Boys**	**Girls**	**Children**
Total	**128**	**1944**	**1041**	**602**	**2107**	**1608**	**3715**	**39.93**	**32.11**	**36.11**
Precursor cell leukaemias	126	1924	1024	585	2063	1596	3659	39.12	31.89	35.59
CD10 positive	32	1453	639	321	1366	1078	2445	26.23	21.70	24.02
Null cell	52	24	27	23	67	59	126	1.29	1.20	1.25
T-cell	6	113	170	110	263	136	399	4.71	2.56	3.66
Other and unspecified	36	334	188	131	367	322	689	6.89	6.42	6.66
Mature B-cell leukaemias	2	19	17	16	42	12	54	0.77	0.23	0.50
B-ALL	2	19	17	16	42	12	54	0.77	0.23	0.50
Lymphoid leukaemia, NOS	0	1	0	1	2	0	2	0.04	0.00	0.02

ASR, age-standardized rate based on World Standard Population

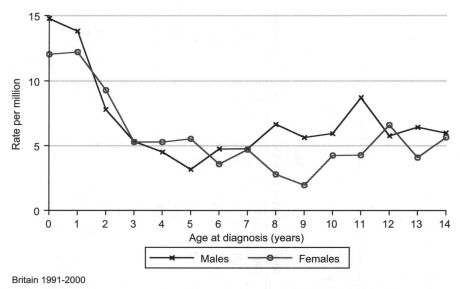

Britain 1991-2000

Fig. 3.12 Annual incidence rates by single year of age for acute myeloid leukaemias (AMLs), by sex, Great Britain, 1991–2000.

and chronic myeloproliferative disease NOS. There were no cases of chronic neutrophilic or eosinophilic leukaemia. The remaining conditions other than CML have been excluded from this study because registration was not felt to be reliable (see Chapter 2), and therefore the diagnostic subgroup is equivalent to CML. Incidence of CML increased with age (Fig. 3.13) and more than half the cases were diagnosed at age 10–14 years and above. The youngest patient in this series was 1 year of age, though CML has occasionally occurred in the first year of life (Boque and Wilson, 1977).

By contrast, the incidence of myelodysplastic syndrome (MDS) and other myeloproliferative diseases decreased with age (Fig. 3.13). About one-third of cases in this subgroup were juvenile myelomonocytic leukaemia (JMML, formerly known as juvenile CML) or chronic myelomonocytic leukaemia (CMML), and two-thirds were MDS (Table 3.5). Incidence of both groups of diseases was highest in infancy. Three-quarters of cases of JMML/CMML were in boys, but there was a small excess of MDS in girls.

Only 1% of leukaemias were of other or unspecified type. Incidence was again highest in infancy. Of the total, 16% were unspecified myeloid leukaemia or chloroma, 59% were acute leukaemia of mixed lymphoid/myeloid or unspecified lineage and the remaining 25% were totally unspecified.

Of the 63 cases coded as CML, 32 (51%) were confirmed as having the Philadelphia chromosome which is characteristic of true, adult-type CML (Chessells, 1992). In a further 16 (25%), there was an explicit statement or other strong evidence that the diagnosis was adult-type CML. Of the remaining 15 children, 12 were aged 10–14 years at diagnosis.

Table 3.4 Numbers of registrations and age-standardized annual incidence per million children for acute myeloid leukaemias (AMLs) by FAB subtype, Great Britain, 1991–2000

Age group (years) at diagnosis	Registrations				Total			ASR		
	0	1–4	5–9	10–14	Boys	Girls	Children	Boys	Girls	Children
	Children									
Total	96	231	161	205	384	309	693	7.10	6.06	6.59
M0	0	3	3	4	5	5	10	0.09	0.10	0.09
M1	1	9	17	26	28	25	53	0.49	0.45	0.47
M2	3	17	39	30	53	36	89	0.94	0.67	0.80
M3	0	18	17	24	32	27	59	0.56	0.52	0.54
M4	14	26	30	29	54	45	99	1.00	0.86	0.93
M5	34	44	13	27	68	50	118	1.32	1.02	1.17
M6	2	3	2	3	5	5	10	0.09	0.11	0.10
M7	18	48	7	4	37	40	77	0.75	0.85	0.80
Unspecified	24	63	33	58	102	76	178	1.88	1.51	1.70

ASR, age-standardized rate based on World Standard Population

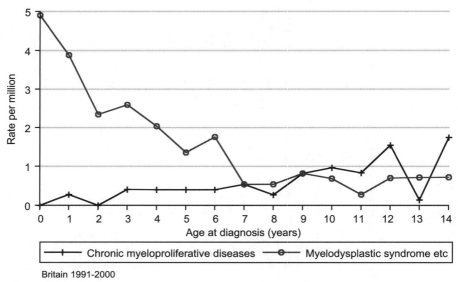

Fig. 3.13 Annual incidence rates by single year of age for myelodysplasia and chronic myeloproliferative diseases, Great Britain, 1991–2000.

The incidence of ALL, like that of all cancers combined, was at the lower end of the range for western countries (Coebergh *et al.*, 2006). The incidence in France, however, was slightly lower than in Britain, with an ASR of 32.3 per million, despite the fact that the French series included no cases of unspecified leukaemia (Clavel *et al.*, 2004). The marked peak of ALL in early childhood is typical of industrialized countries (Stiller and Parkin, 1996; Steliarova-Foucher *et al.*, 2004). In the present series, children aged 1–4 years accounted for 52% of the total cumulative risk of ALL in the first 15 years of life, a similar proportion to that observed in many other western countries (Parkin *et al.*, 1998; Netherlands Cancer Registry, 2000; German Childhood Cancer Registry, 2002; Coebergh *et al.*, 2006). The slightly later peak in incidence for boys compared with girls has also been observed in France (Clavel *et al.*, 2004). The pattern of increasing sex ratio (M:F) with age, from slight excess of girls in the first year of life, followed by male excesses of 1.2:1 at age 1–4 and 1.3:1 at ages 5–9 and 10–14, is continued until at least age 25–29 (Cartwright *et al.*, 2002). Total incidence of ALL was about 10% higher in the Nordic countries in 1990–2001 than the rate for Britain reported here (Hjalgrim *et al.*, 2003). Incidence of T-cell ALL in the Nordic countries was about 3.7 per million (Hjalgrim *et al.*, 2003), very similar to that in Britain. Precursor B-cell ALL, however, had an incidence of about 35 per million (Hjalgrim *et al.*, 2003), which would be about 10% higher than in Britain even if all the British cases of unspecified immunophenotype were in fact precursor B-cell. In France, T-cell ALL had higher incidence, ASR 4.7 per million, whereas the incidence of precursor B-cell ALL, 27.4 per million, was probably somewhat lower than in Britain (Clavel *et al.*, 2004).

Table 3.5 Numbers of registrations and age-standardized annual incidence per million children for myelodysplastic syndrome (MDS) and other myeloproliferative diseases, Great Britain, 1991–2000

Age group (years) at diagnosis	Registrations				Total			ASR		
	0	1–4	5–9	10–14	Boys	Girls	Children	Boys	Girls	Children
	Children									
Total	**35**	**79**	**37**	**22**	**99**	**74**	**173**	**1.94**	**1.50**	**1.72**
JMML and CMML	14	34	6	1	41	14	55	0.83	0.30	0.57
Myelodysplasia	21	45	31	21	58	60	118	1.11	1.20	1.15

ASR, age-standardized rate based on World Standard Population

The incidence of childhood AML in Britain was close to the average for western populations and the age distribution was similar to that seen elsewhere (Smith *et al.*, 1999a; Clavel *et al.*, 2004). The predominance of M2, M4 and M5 was also seen in France (Clavel *et al.*, 2004).

There is hardly any published information on incidence of CML in children, since until recently it was combined in a single diagnostic subgroup with JMML. The detailed diagnostic information available for most cases, together with the predominance of older children, suggest that the great majority of the children registered with CML in this study were correctly classified, though it is of course possible that the subgroup also contains a few cases of JMML/CML. The incidence rate, age distribution and sex ratio for childhood CML in France were similar to those in Britain (Clavel *et al.*, 2004). In Switzerland during 1995–2004, CML accounted for 1.5% of childhood leukaemia (Swiss Childhood Cancer Registry, 2005), a similar proportion to that in Britain.

The incidence of JMML/CMML and MDS was around half that observed in Denmark and British Columbia (Hasle *et al.*, 1995, 1999). Comparison is rendered difficult by varying criteria for the inclusion of cases but it seems likely that the true incidence in the UK is lower than in the other two populations (Passmore *et al.*, 2003). In France, the incidence of JMML/CMML was similar to that in Britain but the rate for MDS was only 0.3 per million (Clavel *et al.*, 2004). In Germany, on the other hand, MDS had a rather higher incidence of 2 per million (German Childhood Cancer Registry, 2002). The excess of boys with JMML/CMML was more pronounced than in the largest published series, where it was 2.1:1 (Niemeyer *et al.*, 1997).

3.3 Lymphomas and reticuloendothelial neoplasms

Lymphomas and reticuloendothelial neoplasms accounted for 9.7% of all registrations. Incidence increased with age (Fig. 3.14), and 18% of cancers at age 10–14 years were lymphomas. Lymphomas were markedly more frequent among boys than girls throughout most of childhood.

Hodgkin lymphomas accounted for 41% of the diagnostic group. They were predominantly cancers of older children. Two-thirds of the cumulative incidence occurred in the 10–14 year age group and there were no registrations at all for infants. Hodgkin lymphomas were almost twice as common among boys as among girls, but the male excess became less marked with increasing age (Fig. 3.15). Histological subtype was specified in 90% of cases (Table 3.6). The most common subtype was nodular sclerosing Hodgkin lymphoma, which accounted for 66% of cases of known subtype. Mixed cellularity accounted for 15%, nodular lymphocyte predominant for 9% and other lymphocyte rich or lymphocyte predominant for 8%. Of the 44 cases in this last category, 16 were specified as lymphocyte-rich classical Hodgkin lymphoma or diffuse lymphocyte predominant and 28 were lymphocyte-predominant NOS, some of which may in fact have been nodular lymphocyte predominant. Lymphocyte-depleted Hodgkin lymphoma was exceedingly rare. Mixed cellularity disease had its peak incidence at age 5–9 years, in contrast to the other main subtypes, whose incidence rose with age. There was an

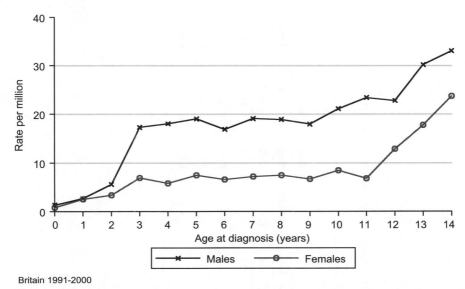

Britain 1991-2000

Fig. 3.14 Annual incidence rates by single year of age for lymphomas and reticuloendothelial neoplasms, by sex, Great Britain, 1991–2000.

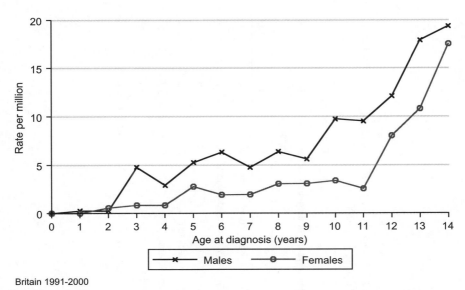

Britain 1991-2000

Fig. 3.15 Annual incidence rates by single year of age for Hodgkin lymphomas, by sex, Great Britain, 1991–2000.

Table 3.6 Numbers of registrations and age-standardized annual incidence per million children for Hodgkin lymphomas by histological subtype, Great Britain, 1991–2000

Age group (years) at diagnosis	Registrations				Total			ASR		
	0	1–4	5–9	10–14	Boys	Girls	Children	Boys	Girls	Children
	Children									
Total	**0**	**39**	**153**	**392**	**385**	**199**	**584**	**6.45**	**3.43**	**4.97**
Nodular lymphocyte predominant	0	4	15	30	38	11	49	0.64	0.20	0.42
Other lymphocyte rich/predominant	0	1	8	35	36	8	44	0.59	0.14	0.37
Mixed cellularity	0	9	38	33	61	19	80	1.04	0.34	0.70
Lymphocyte depleted	0	0	2	2	3	1	4	0.05	0.02	0.03
Nodular sclerosis	0	20	80	251	211	140	351	3.52	2.40	2.97
Unspecified	0	5	10	41	36	20	56	0.61	0.34	0.48

ASR, age-standardized rate based on World Standard Population

excess of boys for all subtypes but this was less marked for nodular sclerosis (M:F = 1.5:1) than for mixed cellularity (3.1:1), nodular lymphocyte predominant (3.2:1) or other lymphocyte rich/predominant (4.2:1). Consequently, nodular sclerosis accounted for a higher proportion of cases of known subtype among girls (78%) than among boys (60%).

NHL, including Burkitt lymphoma, accounted for 57% of lymphomas. NHL was very rare among infants but the incidence increased rather gently through the remainder of childhood (Fig. 3.16). The incidence among boys was over twice that among girls, and the male excess was most marked at age 5–9 years. Out of the total ASR for NHL, 34% was accounted for by mature B-cell (of which 68% were Burkitt lymphomas and 18% were diffuse large-cell lymphomas), 21% by precursor cell and 15% by mature T-cell (Table 3.7). The remaining 29% could not be allocated to any of these categories. As a proportion of the total, B-cell NHL of unknown maturity accounted for 17%, T-cell of unknown maturity for 6% and NHL without specification of lineage or maturity for 6%. Thus, overall 54% of NHL were of B-cell lineage, 40% were T-cell and 6% were unspecified. Precursor cell lymphoma and Burkitt lymphoma had their highest incidence at 5–9 years of age, whereas incidence of other mature B-cell and mature T-cell lymphomas increased with age throughout childhood. The male:female ratio for Burkitt lymphoma was around 4:1 while for the other types it was around 2:1. The majority of mature T-cell lymphomas were anaplastic large-cell lymphoma (ALCL, 73%). The remainder were mycosis fungoides (10%) and other types of peripheral T-cell lymphoma (18%). ALCL was more frequent in boys than girls, and the incidence

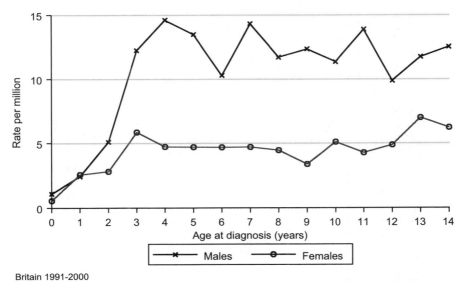

Britain 1991-2000

Fig. 3.16 Annual incidence rates by single year of age for non-Hodgkin lymphomas including Burkitt lymphoma, by sex, Great Britain, 1991–2000.

Table 3.7 Numbers of registrations and age-standardized annual incidence per million children for non-Hodgkin lymphomas (NHLs) (including Burkitt lymphoma) by immunological and histological subtype, Great Britain, 1991–2000

Age group (years) at diagnosis	Registrations				Total			ASR		
	Children				Boys	Girls	Children	Boys	Girls	Children
	0	1–4	5–9	10–14						
Total	**6**	**186**	**313**	**310**	**582**	**233**	**815**	**10.23**	**4.30**	**7.33**
Precursor cell lymphomas	2	48	74	50	117	57	174	2.09	1.07	1.59
Precursor T-cell	1	44	63	45	105	48	153	1.88	0.89	1.40
Precursor B-cell	1	4	11	5	12	9	21	0.21	0.17	0.19
Mature B-cell lymphomas	0	64	100	115	211	68	279	3.70	1.25	2.50
Burkitt lymphoma	0	47	82	62	150	41	191	2.66	0.75	1.73
Other	0	17	18	53	61	27	88	1.04	0.50	0.77
Mature T-cell and NK-cell lymphomas	0	21	43	60	79	45	124	1.36	0.81	1.09
Anaplastic large-cell lymphoma	0	15	29	46	59	31	90	1.01	0.56	0.79
Mycosis fungoides	0	0	4	8	5	7	12	0.08	0.12	0.10
Other	0	6	10	6	15	7	22	0.27	0.13	0.20
Non-Hodgkin lymphomas, NOS	4	53	96	85	175	63	238	3.07	1.18	2.15

ASR, age-standardized rate based on World Standard Population

increased with age. Mycosis fungoides was slightly more frequent in girls and there were no cases diagnosed before the age of 6 years.

Miscellaneous lymphoreticular neoplasms were very rare, accounting for only eight registrations. They comprised five cases of malignant histiocytosis, two of true histiocytic lymphoma and one of malignant mastocytoma. There were also 17 cases of unspecified lymphoma.

There are three main patterns of incidence for childhood Hodgkin lymphomas among mainly white populations of industrialized countries. In Western Europe, Australia and New Zealand, the ASR is often in the range 4–5 per million and around two-thirds of the cumulative incidence is at age 10–14 years (McWhirter et al., 1996; Becroft et al., 1999; Desandes et al., 2004; Clavel et al., 2006). The results reported here are typical of that pattern. In North America the ASR is somewhat higher, about 6 per million, and this is entirely accounted for by higher incidence at age 10–14 years, with three-quarters of the cumulative incidence occurring in this age group (Percy et al., 1999). Finally, Eastern European countries have yet higher incidence, 8–9 per million, and the difference in incidence is particularly marked in earlier childhood, with the cumulative rate for the first 10 years of life in some countries accounting for half of the total (Parkin et al., 1998; Clavel et al., 2006). The decline in sex ratio (M:F) with age continues into adolescence and young adulthood, with males and females having similar incidence at age 15–24 years (Cartwright et al., 2002).

The combined incidence of Burkitt lymphoma and other NHL was typical of western countries (Parkin et al., 1998). While incidence in Britain was slightly higher at age 10–14 years than at age 5–9, however, in most European regions there is a slight peak at age 5–9 (Izarzugaza et al., 2006). In a population-based series of NHL diagnosed at all ages in about 20% of England and Wales, the male excess in adolescence and early adulthood was similar to that reported here for children aged 5–9 and 10–14 (Cartwright et al., 2002); a marked late childhood peak in the sex ratio in that series appears to have been due to an anomalously low incidence among girls aged 10–14 years. The incidence of Burkitt lymphoma was rather low in comparison with that in France (Clavel et al., 2004) and the United States (Percy et al., 1999). This may reflect greater readiness of UK pathologists to classify childhood mature B-cell lymphoma as diffuse large-cell lymphoma rather than Burkitt lymphoma (Lones et al., 2000). As mentioned in Chapter 2, we restricted the inclusion of cases of 'lymphoblastic' lymphoma in the category of precursor cell lymphomas to those which were explicitly described as having T-cell or precursor B-cell immunophenotype, since there is evidence that substantial numbers of Burkitt lymphomas were still being reported as lymphoblastic during the study period (Wright et al., 1997). This will probably have led to an underestimate of the frequency of precursor B-cell NHL. Precursor B-cell disease accounted for a lower proportion of NHL in our study (2.6%) than the 5% in a large series from the Berlin–Frankfurt–Münster (BFM) clinical trials in Germany, Austria and Switzerland (Burkhardt et al., 2005), and the ratio of precursor T-cell to precursor B-cell NHL, 7.3:1, was correspondingly higher than the 3.5:1 in the BFM series. There is no reason to suppose, however, that use of this obsolete term would have differed between the sexes. The sex ratios for

Burkitt lymphoma and other mature B-cell NHL, with a much larger excess of boys with Burkitt lymphoma, were both similar to those found in the BFM series (Burkhardt *et al.*, 2005). The incidence of mycosis fungoides alone in Britain was about 50% higher than that for all cutaneous lymphomas among children in Germany (Stang *et al.*, 2006).

3.4 Summary of lymphoid neoplasms

Table 3.8 summarizes the incidence of lymphoid leukaemias and NHL, including Burkitt lymphoma. Precursor cell malignancies accounted for 85% of the total, mature cell for 10% and unspecified for 5%. B-cell lineage was more frequent than T-cell among both precursor and mature cell neoplasms. Among precursor cell malignancies of both lineages, leukaemia was more frequent than lymphoma, with leukaemia:lymphoma ratios of 2.6:1 for T-cell and more than 100:1 for B-cell. The pattern was reversed for mature cell malignancies: there were no mature T-cell leukaemias at all, and B-cell lymphomas had an incidence rate five times that of B-cell leukaemia. In precursor T-cell disease, the sex ratio and age distributions were similar for leukaemia and lymphoma. The sex ratio of 1.3:1 for precursor B-cell disease was lower than that of 2.6:1 for mature B-cell disease. In both precursor and mature B-cell disease, children with leukaemia tended to be younger than those with lymphoma. The relative frequencies of the different subtypes of lymphoid neoplasms among British children were similar to those in the United States (Morton *et al.*, 2006).

3.5 CNS and miscellaneous intracranial and intraspinal neoplasms

The tumours classified here accounted for 25% of all registrations, making them second in frequency only to the leukaemias overall. The variation in incidence with age was much less than for leukaemia (Fig. 3.17). From age 7 years onwards, the incidence was slightly higher than for leukaemia.

Ependymomas and choroid plexus tumours together accounted for 10% of brain and spinal tumours. Incidence was highest at 1 year of age (Fig. 3.18). In this series, 74% of the subgroup were ependymomas and 26% were choroid plexus tumours (Table 3.9). Ependymoma was most common at age 1–4 years, when its incidence was around twice that in older age groups. Below 10 years of age there was a male excess but this was reversed at age 10–14. The primary site for ependymoma was the brain in 88% of cases and the spinal cord in 11% (Table 3.10). There were also two children with extradural sacrococcygeal primary site. Among ependymomas of the brain with specified, non-ventricular site, 75% were infratentorial and 25% were supratentorial. Spinal cord ependymomas were very rare in early childhood, with 93% of cases occurring at age 5–14 years. The proportions of different primary sites were fairly similar in boys and girls. Anaplastic ependymoma or ependymoblastoma accounted for 20% of all ependymomas, myxopapillary ependymoma for 6.5%, subependymoma for 2.7% and papillary ependymoma for 1.9%; the remaining 69% were not of any specified subtype. Although ependymoma overall was most frequent among young children,

Table 3.8 Numbers of registrations and age-standardized annual incidence per million children for lymphoid leukaemias and non-Hodgkin lymphomas (NHLs) (including Burkitt lymphoma) by cell lineage and maturity, Great Britain, 1991–2000

Age group (years) at diagnosis			Registrations							ASR		
			Children				Total					
Maturity	Lineage		0	1–4	5–9	10–14	Boys	Girls	Children	Boys	Girls	Children
Precursor cell	Total	Leukaemia	126	1924	1024	585	2063	1596	3659	39.12	31.89	35.59
		Lymphoma	2	48	74	50	117	57	174	2.09	1.07	1.59
	B-cell	Leukaemia	85	1477	668	344	1436	1138	2574	27.58	22.90	25.29
		Lymphoma	1	4	11	5	12	9	21	0.21	0.17	0.19
	T-cell	Leukaemia	6	113	170	110	263	136	399	4.71	2.56	3.66
		Lymphoma	1	44	63	45	105	48	153	1.88	0.89	1.40
	Unspecified	Leukaemia	35	334	186	131	364	322	686	6.84	6.42	6.63
		Lymphoma	0	0	0	0	0	0	0	0.00	0.00	0.00
Mature cell	Total	Leukaemia	2	19	17	16	42	12	54	0.77	0.23	0.50
		Lymphoma	0	85	143	175	290	113	403	5.07	2.05	3.59
	B-cell	Leukaemia	2	19	17	16	42	12	54	0.77	0.23	0.50
		Lymphoma	0	64	100	115	211	68	279	3.70	1.25	2.50
	T-cell	Leukaemia	0	0	0	0	0	0	0	0.00	0.00	0.00
		Lymphoma	0	21	43	60	79	45	124	1.36	0.81	1.09
Unspecified	Total	Leukaemia	0	1	0	1	2	0	2	0.04	0.00	0.02
		Lymphoma	4	53	96	85	175	63	238	3.07	1.18	2.15
	B-cell	Leukaemia	0	0	0	0	0	0	0	0.00	0.00	0.00
		Lymphoma	2	30	52	54	108	30	138	1.90	0.55	1.24
	T-cell	Leukaemia	0	0	0	0	0	0	0	0.00	0.00	0.00
		Lymphoma	0	11	23	15	35	14	49	0.61	0.27	0.44
	Unspecified	Leukaemia	0	1	0	1	2	0	2	0.04	0.00	0.02
		Lymphoma	2	12	21	16	32	19	51	0.57	0.36	0.46

ASR, age-standardized rate based on World Standard Population

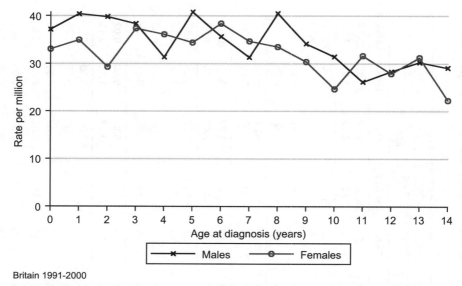

Britain 1991-2000

Fig. 3.17 Annual incidence rates by single year of age for CNS and miscellaneous intracranial and intraspinal neoplasms, by sex, Great Britain, 1991–2000.

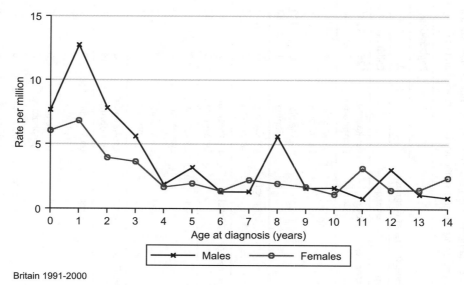

Britain 1991-2000

Fig. 3.18 Annual incidence rates by single year of age for ependymomas and choroid plexus tumours, by sex, Great Britain, 1991–2000.

Table 3.9 Numbers of registrations and age-standardized annual incidence per million children for ependymomas and choroid plexus tumour, Great Britain, 1991–2000

Age group (years) at diagnosis	Registrations				Total			ASR		
	0	1–4	5–9	10–14	Boys	Girls	Children	Boys	Girls	Children
	Children									
Total	**49**	**161**	**82**	**60**	**208**	**144**	**352**	**4.03**	**2.85**	**3.45**
Ependymomas	13	121	71	56	146	115	261	2.77	2.23	2.51
Choroid plexus tumour	36	40	11	4	62	29	91	1.25	0.62	0.95
Papilloma	20	20	8	3	32	19	51	0.64	0.40	0.52
Carcinoma	16	20	3	1	30	10	40	0.61	0.22	0.42

ASR, age-standardized rate based on World Standard Population

Table 3.10 Numbers of registrations and age-standardized annual incidence per million children for ependymomas by primary site, Great Britain, 1991–2000

Age group (years) at diagnosis	Registrations				Total			ASR		
	Children				Boys	Girls	Children	Boys	Girls	Children
	0	1–4	5–9	10–14						
Total	**13**	**121**	**71**	**56**	**146**	**115**	**261**	**2.77**	**2.23**	**2.51**
Supratentorial brain	1	16	19	11	24	23	47	0.44	0.44	0.44
Cerebellum	9	88	24	14	79	56	135	1.57	1.14	1.36
Brain stem	0	3	4	2	4	5	9	0.08	0.09	0.08
Ventricles	2	10	7	5	15	9	24	0.28	0.18	0.23
Other and unspecified brain	1	2	5	6	5	9	14	0.09	0.16	0.13
Spinal cord	0	2	11	17	18	12	30	0.30	0.21	0.26
Extradural	0	0	1	1	1	1	2	0.02	0.02	0.02

ASR, age-standardized rate based on World Standard Population

all cases of the myxopapillary subtype were diagnosed at 5–14 years of age. The primary site of myxopapillary ependymoma was the spinal cord in 12/17 (71%) cases, and the two extradural ependymomas were also of this subtype. Among the choroid plexus tumours, benign papillomas were slightly more frequent than malignant carcinomas (Table 3.9). Choroid plexus tumours had their highest incidence in infancy and there was a male excess of 2.0:1 overall, 1.6:1 for papilloma and 2.8:1 for carcinoma.

Astrocytomas were the most common brain and spinal neoplasms, over 40% of the total. Incidence was slightly higher at ages 1–9 years than among infants or older children (Fig. 3.19). There was a small female excess, and no consistent variation in the sex ratio with age. Astrocytomas encompass a wide range of behaviour, from the low-grade pilocytic (juvenile) astrocytoma to the highly aggressive glioblastoma multiforme (Table 3.11). In this series, 76% of astrocytomas were low grade (WHO Grade 1 or 2), 15% were high grade (WHO 3 or 4) and 9% were of unspecified grade. Children with low-grade astrocytomas tended to be younger than those with high grade, though the highest frequency of both groups occurred in the 5–9 year age range. The primary site for astrocytoma was intracranial in 95% of cases and the spinal cord in 5% (Table 3.12); there were also two cases of retinal astrocytoma. Among intracranial astrocytomas of specified, non-ventricular site, 30% were cerebral, 39% were cerebellar, 14% were in the brain stem and 17% were in the optic pathway. Cerebral tumours had a peak of incidence in infancy; their incidence then fell at age 1–4 years before increasing through the remainder of childhood. Infratentorial tumours of both cerebellum and brain stem were most common at age 5–9 years and optic nerve tumours at age

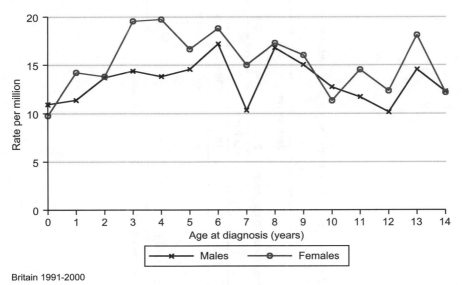

Britain 1991-2000

Fig. 3.19 Annual incidence rates by single year of age for astrocytomas, by sex, Great Britain, 1991–2000.

Table 3.11 Numbers of registrations and age-standardized annual incidence per million children for astrocytomas by WHO grade, Great Britain, 1991–2000

Age group (years) at diagnosis	Registrations					Total			ASR		
	Children	0	1–4	5–9	10–14	Boys	Girls	Children	Boys	Girls	Children
Total	**74**	**439**	**579**	**459**		**739**	**812**	**1551**	**13.31**	**15.36**	**14.31**
Grades 1–2	60	359	441	319		557	622	1179	10.10	11.85	10.95
Grades 3–4	11	52	95	80		116	122	238	2.06	2.27	2.16
Unspecified grade	3	28	43	60		66	68	134	1.16	1.24	1.20

ASR, age-standardized rate based on World Standard Population

Table 3.12 Numbers of registrations and age-standardized annual incidence per million children for astrocytomas by primary site, Great Britain, 1991–2000

Age group (years) at diagnosis	Registrations (Children)				Total			ASR		
	0	1–4	5–9	10–14	Boys	Girls	Children	Boys	Girls	Children
Total	**74**	**439**	**579**	**459**	**739**	**812**	**1551**	**13.31**	**15.36**	**14.31**
Supratentorial brain	31	79	127	152	195	194	389	3.48	3.59	3.54
Cerebellum	3	156	209	136	236	268	504	4.23	5.07	4.64
Brain stem	2	45	84	49	91	89	180	1.62	1.66	1.64
Ventricles	5	12	22	32	34	37	71	0.59	0.69	0.64
Other and unspecified brain	7	25	38	46	54	62	116	0.96	1.15	1.05
Optic nerves	21	90	77	26	96	118	214	1.83	2.33	2.07
Spinal cord	4	31	22	18	32	43	75	0.59	0.84	0.71
Retina	1	1	0	0	1	1	2	0.02	0.02	0.02

ASR, age-standardized rate based on World Standard Population

1–4 years. In contrast to spinal cord ependymomas, astrocytomas of this site were most frequent at age 1–4 years.

Intracranial and intraspinal embryonal tumours were most frequent in early childhood (Fig. 3.20). Incidence declined gently with age until around 9 years, and more steeply thereafter. There was a male excess which was more pronounced than for any other subgroup of intracranial and intraspinal tumours. The sex ratio increased with age, from 1.1:1 in infancy to 2.1:1 at age 10–14. Nearly three-quarters of the subgroup were medulloblastomas, i.e. primitive neuroectodermal tumours (PNETs) of the cerebellum (Table 3.13). Medulloblastoma was most frequent at age 5–9 years, and the sex ratio was 1.6:1. Other PNET tended to occur more often in younger children; the highest incidence was in infancy, and 59% of registrations were for children under 5 years of age. In contrast to medulloblastoma, there was only a small male excess for other PNET. Nearly all the remainder of the subgroup were atypical teratoid/rhabdoid tumours (ATRTs). Incidence was highest in infancy, and 75% of registrations were for children below the age of 5 years. ATRT occurred in equal numbers among boys and girls. Of the 24 registered cases, 23 (96%) were intracranial and 1 was in the spinal cord. Intracranial ATRT of specified non-ventricular sites was slightly more frequent in supratentorial sites (56%) than infratentorial (44%).

The great majority (86%) of the subgroup of other gliomas were unspecified gliomas (Table 3.14); of these, histological verification was recorded for only 22%. There was a pronounced peak of incidence at age 5–9 years, and boys and girls had similar incidence. By far the most frequent primary site (214/328, 65%) was the brain stem. Nearly all

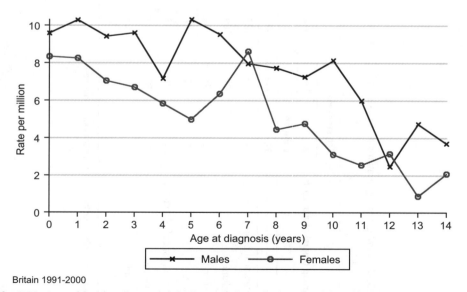

Britain 1991-2000

Fig. 3.20 Annual incidence rates by single year of age for intracranial and intraspinal embryonal tumours, by sex, Great Britain, 1991–2000.

Table 3.13 Numbers of registrations and age-standardized annual incidence per million children for intracranial and intraspinal embryonal tumours, Great Britain, 1991–2000

Age group (years) at diagnosis	Registrations				Total			ASR		
	Children				Boys	Girls	Children	Boys	Girls	Children
	0	1–4	5–9	10–14						
Total	64	235	266	132	423	274	697	7.79	5.37	6.61
Medulloblastomas	29	156	221	103	322	187	509	5.87	3.59	4.76
Primitive neuroectodermal tumour (PNET)	27	68	40	26	87	74	161	1.65	1.50	1.58
Medulloepithelioma	0	1	2	0	2	1	3	0.03	0.02	0.03
Atypical teratoid/rhabdoid tumour	8	10	3	3	12	12	24	0.23	0.25	0.24

ASR, age-standardized rate based on World Standard Population

Table 3.14 Numbers of registrations and age-standardized annual incidence per million children for other gliomas, Great Britain, 1991–2000

Age group (years) at diagnosis	Registrations				Total			ASR		
	0	1–4	5–9	10–14	Boys	Girls	Children	Boys	Girls	Children
	Children									
Total	**14**	**93**	**166**	**107**	**192**	**188**	**380**	**3.45**	**3.50**	**3.47**
Oligodendrogliomas	1	6	7	18	17	15	32	0.30	0.27	0.28
Mixed and unspecified gliomas	12	86	158	87	172	171	343	3.10	3.19	3.14
Mixed gliomas	0	2	9	4	6	9	15	0.11	0.16	0.13
Unspecified gliomas	12	84	149	83	166	162	328	3.00	3.03	3.01
Neuroepithelial glial tumours of uncertain origin	1	1	1	2	3	2	5	0.05	0.04	0.05

ASR, age-standardized rate based on World Standard Population

remaining cases in the subgroup were mixed gliomas and oligodendrogliomas. Oligodendroglioma occurred with similar frequency among boys and girls, and more than half the cases were in children aged 10–14 years. Nearly all (27/29, 93%) oligodendrogliomas of specified site were supratentorial. Eight (25%) of the oligodendrogliomas were specified as anaplastic or oligodendroblastoma.

The miscellaneous subgroup of other specified intracranial and intraspinal neoplasms comprises pituitary adenoma and carcinoma, craniopharyngioma, pineal parenchymal tumours, neuronal and mixed neuronal–glial tumours and meningioma (Table 3.15). Pituitary adenoma and carcinoma were hardly ever diagnosed before the age of 10 years. Craniopharyngioma was the most common tumour within the subgroup; incidence was higher at age 5 years and above and there was a male excess (sex ratio 1.2:1). The majority (27/38, 71%) of pineal parenchymal tumours were pineoblastomas. Of the remainder, 9 (24%) were pineocytomas and 2 (5%) were pinealomas. Pineoblastoma was equally frequent in the two sexes, and two-thirds of cases were diagnosed in the first 5 years of life. The sex ratio and age distribution were thus quite similar to those for supratentorial PNET, with which pineoblastoma is sometimes classified (Pizer *et al.*, 2006). Pineocytoma, by contrast, was predominantly seen in the 10–14 age group and six of the nine cases were in boys. Almost half (49%) of the neuronal and neuronal–glial tumours were gangliogliomas, 44% were dysembryoplastic neuroepithelial tumours (DNET) and 8% were central neurocytomas. Desmoplastic infantile ganglioglioma occurred almost exclusively in infants, though there was one case in a child aged 2 years; boys were affected more than three times as often as girls. Other gangliogliomas had fairly constant incidence throughout childhood and there was a female excess (sex ratio 0.64:1). DNET was rare before the age of 5 years. It was more frequent among boys than girls (sex ratio 1.6:1). Incidence of meningioma increased throughout childhood, more than half of the registrations being at age 10–14, and there was a male excess (sex ratio 1.5:1).

Finally, unspecified tumours accounted for 5% of the group of intracranial and intraspinal neoplasms. The great majority (85%) were unverified histologically. Incidence was highest in infancy, and there was a slight excess of boys. Ill-defined and unspecified sites in the brain accounted for 43% of cases.

Table 3.16 shows the overall distribution of tumour types by site within the brain and spinal cord. These data include not only all registrations in the diagnostic group of CNS and miscellaneous intracranial and intraspinal neoplasms, but also those from other groups or subgroups; five registrations for CNS tumours not specified as between brain and spinal cord have been omitted. Overall, 90% of the total was accounted for by specified tumour types within the group of intracranial and intraspinal neoplasms, 5% by specified tumours of other diagnostic groups and 5% by unspecified tumours. One-third of all the tumours of specified type were low-grade astrocytomas, high-grade and unspecified astrocytomas together accounted for a further 10%, and other and unspecified gliomas for 10%. In total, 53% of specified tumours were gliomas. Medulloblastoma and other PNET accounted for 18%, ependymoma for 7%, craniopharyngioma for 5%, germ cell tumours for 5%, and a wide range of other tumours for the remaining 11%. Unspecified neoplasms accounted for under 10% of tumours in

Table 3.15 Numbers of registrations and age-standardized annual incidence per million children for other specified intracranial and intraspinal neoplasms, Great Britain, 1991–2000

Age group (years) at diagnosis	Registrations (Children)				Total			ASR		
	0	1–4	5–9	10–14	Boys	Girls	Children	Boys	Girls	Children
Total	**28**	**81**	**158**	**185**	**253**	**199**	**452**	**4.45**	**3.67**	**4.07**
Pituitary adenomas and carcinomas	0	1	1	21	13	10	23	0.21	0.17	0.19
Tumours of the sellar region (craniopharyngiomas)	5	34	83	79	114	87	201	1.98	1.59	1.79
Pineal parenchymal tumours	5	15	8	10	21	17	38	0.39	0.34	0.37
Neuronal and mixed neuronal–glial tumours	17	23	53	49	75	67	142	1.35	1.24	1.30
Desmoplastic infantile ganglioglioma	8	1	0	0	7	2	9	0.15	0.04	0.10
Other ganglioglioma	6	12	21	21	24	36	60	0.43	0.67	0.55
Dysembryoplastic neuroepithelial tumour	3	8	26	25	38	24	62	0.67	0.43	0.55
Central neurocytoma	0	2	6	3	6	5	11	0.10	0.09	0.10
Meningiomas	1	8	13	26	30	18	48	0.51	0.33	0.42

ASR, age-standardized rate based on World Standard Population

Table 3.16 Numbers of registrations for intracranial and intraspinal neoplasms by histological type and primary site, Great Britain, 1991–2000

Histological type	Primary site										Total
	Supratentorial brain	Cerebellum	Brain stem	Ventricles	Other and unspecified brain	Pituitary and sellar	Pineal	Optic and cranial nerves	Spinal cord	Meninges	
Ependymomas	47	135	9	24	13	0	0	0	30	0	258
Choroid plexus tumour	1	2	0	87	1	0	0	0	0	0	91
Astrocytoma grades 1–2	220	461	83	60	81	0	3	214	55	1	1178
Astrocytoma grades 3–4	134	15	65	4	9	0	0	0	11	0	238
Unspecified astrocytoma	30	28	32	7	24	1	1	0	8	2	133
Medulloblastomas	0	502	0	5	2	0	0	0	0	0	509
Primitive neuroectodermal tumour (PNET)	85	37	4	10	12	0	4	0	6	2	160
Atypical teratoid/rhabdoid tumour	9	8	0	3	2	0	1	0	1	0	24
Oligodendrogliomas	27	2	0	0	3	0	0	0	0	0	32
Other and unspecified glioma	82	8	214	3	27	0	2	5	5	0	346
Pituitary adenomas and carcinomas	0	0	0	0	0	23	0	0	0	0	23
Tumours of the sellar region (craniopharyngiomas)	1	0	0	0	0	198	0	0	0	0	199
Pineal parenchymal tumours	0	0	0	0	0	0	38	0	0	0	38
Ganglioglioma	45	6	4	0	8	0	0	1	4	0	68
Dysembryoplastic neuroepithelial tumour	59	0	0	0	3	0	0	0	0	0	62

Table 3.16 (continued) Numbers of registrations for intracranial and intraspinal neoplasms by histological type and primary site, Great Britain, 1991–2000

Histological type	Primary site										
	Supratentorial brain	Cerebellum	Brain stem	Ventricles	Other and unspecified brain	Pituitary and sellar	Pineal	Optic and cranial nerves	Spinal cord	Meninges	Total
Other specified CNS tumours	5	2	0	3	3	0	0	0	1	0	14
Meningiomas	5	2	0	6	3	0	0	2	0	27	45
Malignant germ cell tumours	20	5	0	8	21	11	61	2	0	0	128
Other and unspecified germ cell tumours	5	0	1	4	13	0	6	0	7	0	36
Lymphoma	3	2	1	0	2	0	0	0	1	0	9
Neuroblastoma and ganglioneuroblastoma	2	0	0	0	1	0	0	0	1	0	4
Paraganglioma	0	0	0	0	0	0	0	0	0	1	1
Sarcoma	3	3	0	0	5	0	0	1	3	1	16
Melanoma	2	0	0	1	0	0	0	0	1	5	9
Unspecified tumours	30	17	21	5	69	9	8	5	4	4	172
Total	815	1235	434	230	302	242	124	230	138	43	3793

all site groups except ill-defined and unspecified brain. The distribution of specified tumour types varied markedly between sites. Several tumour types occurred in supratentorial brain sites with reasonable frequency, the most numerous being low-grade astrocytoma (28%), high-grade astrocytoma (17%), other gliomas including unspecified astrocytoma and oligodendroglioma (18%), PNET (11%), DNET (8%), ependymoma (6%) and ganglioglioma (6%). Cerebellar tumours were predominantly medulloblastoma and other PNET (44%), low-grade astrocytoma (38%), and ependymoma (11%); in contrast to supratentorial sites, high-grade astrocytoma was very unusual in the cerebellum. Among brain stem tumours, 44% were astrocytoma, with low grade slightly more frequent than high grade, and 52% were other gliomas, mostly not otherwise specified. By far the most frequent tumour of the pituitary/sellar region in childhood was craniopharyngioma (85%). Over half (58%) of pineal tumours of specified type were germ-cell tumours, and just under one-third (33%) were pineal parenchymal tumours. The vast majority (95%) of optic and cranial nerve tumours were low-grade astrocytomas. In the spinal cord, 55% of tumours were astrocytomas and 22% were ependymomas.

Some of the largest international variations in recorded incidence of childhood cancer between western countries relate to intracranial and intraspinal tumours (Parkin et al., 1998; Stiller et al., 2006b). This is partly accounted for by differences in registration practice. Until recently, most cancer registries in North America have not registered non-malignant CNS tumours, and it has been estimated that this has caused a shortfall of 18% in total recorded incidence among children (Gurney et al., 1999d). In some countries, also, there have been particular difficulties in ascertaining CNS tumours (Kaatsch et al., 2001). It is reasonable to suspect that any under registration disproportionately affects lower grade and non-malignant tumours, since children with these diagnoses would tend to visit fewer departments in the course of treatment for the one tumour, providing correspondingly fewer opportunities for registration. Total incidence of CNS tumours in Britain was somewhat higher than in most parts of Europe apart from the Nordic countries, where rates have been comparatively high since at least the late 1970s (Peris-Bonet et al., 2006).

Incidence rates for ependymoma and choroid plexus tumours combined were similar to those from other registries. The age distribution for ependymomas was similar to that in the United States (Gurney et al., 1999a; CBTRUS, 2002). Incidence of choroid plexus papilloma was comparable with that in the CBTRUS (Gurney et al., 1999d).

Astrocytoma is not only the most frequent childhood CNS tumour but also shows a very wide range of reported incidence, even from registries in western countries with good completeness of ascertainment. The ASR for Great Britain was similar to those in many European countries (Parkin et al., 1998; Peris-Bonet et al., 2006) and the United States (Gurney et al., 1999a). The absence of any marked variation in incidence with age is usual for this tumour, irrespective of the total incidence rate (Parkin et al., 1998). The predominance of low-grade tumours was similar to that observed in Germany (Kaatsch et al., 2001) and the United States (CBTRUS, 2002).

Incidence rates for embryonal tumours, predominantly medulloblastoma and other PNET, were similar to those from other registries (Gurney *et al.*, 1999a; Peris-Bonet *et al.*, 2006). The ratio of medulloblastoma to other PNET was similar to that in Germany (Kaatsch *et al.*, 2001). The United States SEER registries also had a greater proportion of boys with medulloblastoma compared to other PNET (McNeil *et al.*, 2002). For ATRT, the predominance of young children and a predilection for supratentorial sites were also found in a United States multi-centre clinical series (Hilden *et al.*, 2004). The equal representation of the two sexes in our series, however, contrasts with the excess of boys (2:1) in the American series. Patterns of incidence for rhabdoid tumours of all primary sites combined are presented after the section on soft tissue sarcomas below.

Incidence of craniopharyngioma was comparable with that reported from the United States (Bunin *et al.*, 1998; Gurney *et al.*, 1999d; CBTRUS, 2002), Germany (Kaatsch *et al.*, 2001) and Europe as a whole (Peris-Bonet *et al.*, 2006). The age distribution and sex ratio were similar to those in the United States (Bunin *et al.*, 1998). Incidence has rarely been reported for the other entities in the subgroup of other specified intracranial and intraspinal neoplasms; the rates reported here are similar to those for Europe as a whole (Peris-Bonet *et al.*, 2006). Judging by the CBTRUS data (Gurney *et al.*, 1999d), incidence rates are rather higher in the United States for meningioma (0.6 per million) and pituitary tumours (0.4 per million).

3.6 Neuroblastoma and other peripheral nervous cell tumours

By far the most common malignant tumour in this group was neuroblastoma, including ganglioneuroblastoma, which accounted for 6% of all cancers and was the most common of the four principal embryonal tumours of childhood. The incidence was highest in infancy and declined sharply beyond the age of 5 years (Fig. 3.21). Neuroblastoma was the most frequent single type of cancer in the first year of life, accounting for 19% of all cancers in infants. The incidence was higher among boys, with a male:female ratio of 1.2:1. The male excess was fairly constant throughout childhood (Fig. 3.22). Almost one-half (46%) of neuroblastoma had the adrenal gland as primary site (Table 3.17), with retroperitoneal and other abdominal primaries accounting for a further 26% and thoracic sites for 13%. Nearly all the remainder were in other or ill-specified sites in the trunk or of unknown primary site, but 3% were in head and neck sites. There was little variation in age or sex between primary sites except for the especially high proportion of infants in the small group of head and neck primaries and the slight excess of girls with thoracic neuroblastoma. There were only 11 registrations of other peripheral nervous cell tumours; of these, 5 were olfactory neuroblastoma and 3 were malignant paraganglioma.

The incidence of neuroblastoma was somewhat lower than in many other industrialized countries (Parkin *et al.*, 1998; Goodman *et al.*, 1999; Spix *et al.*, 2006). The deficit was most marked during the first year of life. In Japan, where there was until recently a national screening programme for neuroblastoma, and in parts of some other countries where screening was undertaken as a research project, the excess can be explained by the

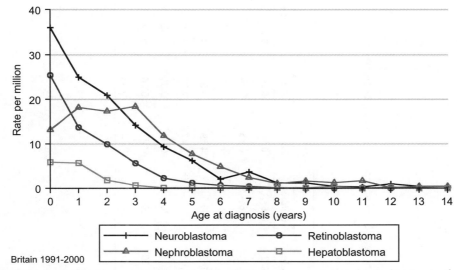

Britain 1991-2000

Fig. 3.21 Annual incidence rates by single year of age for the principal embryonal tumours of childhood, Great Britain, 1991–2000.

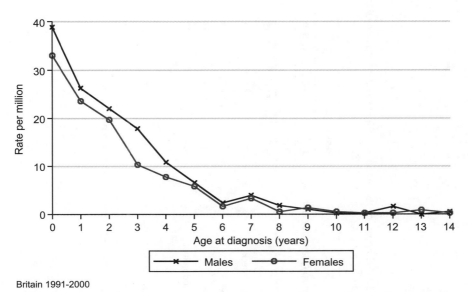

Britain 1991-2000

Fig. 3.22 Annual incidence rates by single year of age for neuroblastoma and ganglioneuroblastoma, by sex, Great Britain, 1991–2000.

Table 3.17 Numbers of registrations and age-standardized annual incidence per million children for neuroblastoma and ganglioneuroblastoma by primary site, Great Britain, 1991–2000

Age group (years) at diagnosis	Registrations				Total			ASR		
	0	1–4	5–9	10–14	Boys	Girls	Children	Boys	Girls	Children
	Children									
Total	257	505	106	18	499	387	886	10.16	8.26	9.23
Head and neck	13	11	4	0	17	11	28	0.35	0.24	0.29
Thoracic	44	56	13	2	55	60	115	1.11	1.30	1.20
Adrenal	123	233	48	5	240	169	409	4.89	3.62	4.27
Other abdominal	43	147	28	9	122	105	227	2.47	2.22	2.34
Pelvic	10	17	3	0	16	14	30	0.33	0.30	0.32
Other and unspecified trunk	6	13	3	1	13	10	23	0.27	0.20	0.24
Unspecified	18	28	7	1	36	18	54	0.73	0.38	0.56

ASR, age-standardized rate based on World Standard Population

detection of large numbers of tumours that would otherwise have remained asymptomatic (Ajiki *et al.*, 1998; Schilling *et al.*, 2002; Honjo *et al.*, 2003). The recorded incidence in infancy has still been higher in the United States and many European countries than in Britain (Goodman *et al.*, 1999; Spix *et al.*, 2006) and it has been suggested that this may reflect increased detection of neuroblastoma by informal screening (Goodman *et al.*, 1999), for example during routine health checks (Powell *et al.*, 1998).

3.7 **Retinoblastoma**

Retinoblastoma is another of the principal embryonal tumours of childhood. Over 40% of the incidence occurred within the first year of life (Fig. 3.21). Overall, males and females had similar incidence. Retinoblastoma was more common among boys in the first year of life and among girls in the second year (Fig. 3.23).

Retinoblastoma was bilateral in 35% of cases and unilateral in 63% (Table 3.18); there was no record of laterality in the remaining 2%. Unilateral and bilateral retinoblastoma both had their highest incidence in the first year of life (Fig. 3.24). The early peak was especially marked for bilateral cases, with 68% diagnosed among infants compared with 29% of unilateral cases. There was a male excess among children with bilateral retinoblastoma, M:F = 1.26:1, whereas unilateral retinoblastoma occurred more often in girls, M:F = 0.85:1.

The incidence and age distribution for retinoblastoma were similar to those observed in other western countries (Parkin *et al.*, 1998; Young *et al.*, 1999). The variations in sex ratio by laterality and between the first and second years of life have also been found

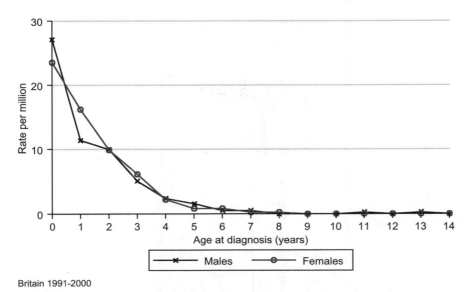

Britain 1991-2000

Fig. 3.23 Annual incidence rates by single year of age for retinoblastoma, by sex, Great Britain, 1991–2000.

Table 3.18 Numbers of registrations and age-standardized annual incidence per million children for retinoblastoma by laterality, Great Britain, 1991–2000

Age group (years) at diagnosis	Registrations				Total			ASR		
	0	1–4	5–9	10–14	Boys	Girls	Children	Boys	Girls	Children
	Children									
Total	**181**	**229**	**18**	**2**	**218**	**212**	**430**	**4.52**	**4.62**	**4.57**
Unilateral	78	174	18	2	129	143	272	2.65	3.10	2.87
Bilateral	103	48	0	0	86	65	151	1.81	1.44	1.63
Unknown laterality	0	7	0	0	3	4	7	0.06	0.09	0.07

ASR, age-standardized rate based on World Standard Population

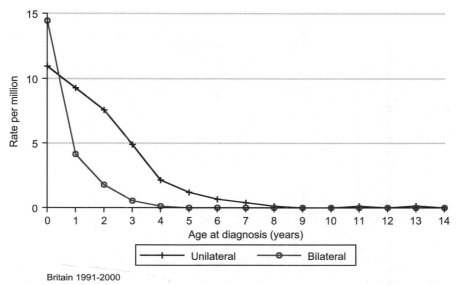

Fig. 3.24 Annual incidence rates by single year of age for retinoblastoma, by laterality
Great Britain, 1991–2000.

in a large series from Europe (MacCarthy *et al.*, 2006). Consistent with Knudson's
two-hit model (Knudson, 1971), retinoblastoma occurs as a result of two mutations
in the retinoblastoma suppressor gene *RB1* and is heritable when the first mutation is
in the germline and non-heritable when both mutations are somatic. Bilateral cases
and those with a positive family history are classified as heritable and the remainder as
non-heritable, though the latter group will include a few undetected children with the
germline mutation. In a study of NRCT cases diagnosed up to 1985, 8% of unilateral
cases had a family history and were therefore heritable (Draper *et al.*, 1992). This suggests
that about 40% of retinoblastoma in the present series were heritable.

3.8 Renal tumours

Nearly all childhood renal tumours were in the subgroup nephroblastoma and other
nonepithelial renal tumours. The great majority, 90% of all renal tumours, were
nephroblastoma (Wilms tumour) (Table 3.19). The peak incidence of nephroblastoma
was at 1–3 years, slightly later than for the other embryonal tumours of childhood
(Fig. 3.21). The two sexes were affected equally, but the peak incidence was at a later
age in girls than in boys (Fig. 3.25). While bilateral nephroblastoma does occur, it is
much rarer than bilateral retinoblastoma. In this series, only 7% of children with
nephroblastoma had bilateral tumours, 90% were unilateral and 3% were of unknown
laterality. As with retinoblastoma, bilateral cases were diagnosed earlier than unilateral
(Fig. 3.26). Infants aged under a year accounted for 29% of bilateral cases and 12%
of unilateral. Incidence of bilateral nephroblastoma was highest in infancy, whereas

Table 3.19 Numbers of registrations and age-standardized annual incidence per million children for nephroblastoma and other nonepithelial renal tumours, Great Britain, 1991–2000

Age group (years) at diagnosis	Registrations					Total			ASR		
	0	1–4	5–9	10–14		Boys	Girls	Children	Boys	Girls	Children
	Children										
Nephroblastoma and other nonepithelial renal tumours	**111**	**506**	**139**	**31**		**400**	**387**	**787**	**8.00**	**8.11**	**8.05**
Nephroblastoma	94	479	131	28		362	370	732	7.23	7.76	7.49
Unilateral	79	429	126	27		334	327	661	6.65	6.84	6.74
Bilateral	15	35	2	0		18	34	52	0.37	0.74	0.55
Unknown laterality	0	15	3	1		10	9	19	0.21	0.18	0.19
Rhabdoid renal tumour	14	10	0	0		17	7	24	0.36	0.15	0.26
Kidney sarcomas	2	17	5	0		18	6	24	0.36	0.13	0.25
Peripheral neuroectodermal tumour (pPNET) of kidney	1	0	3	3		3	4	7	0.05	0.07	0.06

ASR, age-standardized rate based on World Standard Population

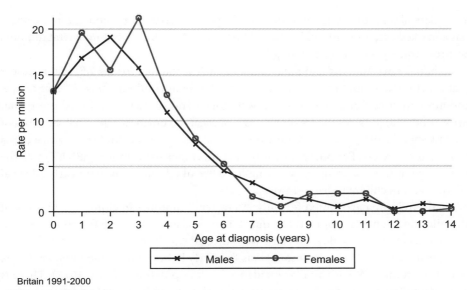

Britain 1991-2000

Fig. 3.25 Annual incidence rates by single year of age for nephroblastoma (Wilms tumour), by sex, Great Britain, 1991–2000.

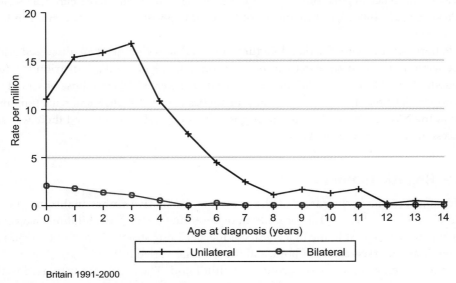

Britain 1991-2000

Fig. 3.26 Annual incidence rates by single year of age for nephroblastoma (Wilms tumour), by laterality, Great Britain, 1991–2000.

for unilateral cases the peak was at the age of 3 years. In contrast to retinoblastoma, there was a marked excess of girls with bilateral tumours (M:F = 0.5:1), but unilateral tumours occurred equally often in boys and girls.

Rhabdoid renal tumour and renal sarcoma each accounted for 3% of renal tumours (Table 3.19). Rhabdoid renal tumour occurred only in children below 5 years of age, and more than half of all registrations were for infants. Boys were affected more than twice as often as girls. All the registered cases of renal sarcoma were clear cell sarcomas of the kidney (CCSK). CCSK was most frequent at age 1–4 years and there was again a marked male excess. Peripheral primitive neuroectodermal tumour (pPNET) was the rarest type in this subgroup, accounting for 0.9% of all renal cancers; nearly all renal pPNET were in children aged 5–14 years.

Renal carcinoma accounted for only 2% of renal tumours in children and 0.1% of all childhood cancers. About three-quarters of registrations were for children aged 10–14 years at diagnosis. Boys and girls were affected equally often.

Nephroblastoma (Wilms tumour) was formerly believed by some to be an 'index cancer of childhood', with similar incidence in all populations (Innis, 1972). There is now known to be considerable international variation, with higher incidence in some black populations in Africa and elsewhere, and lower rates throughout much of Asia (Stiller and Parkin, 1990). The incidence rates reported here were slightly lower than in many western populations (Bernstein *et al.*, 1999a; Pastore *et al.*, 2006b). The deficit was more marked in the first year of life, raising the question of whether there is uniform reporting and registration of malignant nephroblastoma and non-malignant mesoblastic nephroma among infants. Girls in the United States National Wilms' Tumor Study (NWTS) were on average about 6 months older than boys (Breslow *et al.*, 1988). The later peak of incidence in girls compared with boys was also found in a large European series (Pastore *et al.*, 2006b), but incidence of bilateral nephroblastoma was similar in the two sexes.

Patterns of incidence for rhabdoid tumours of all sites combined are discussed after the section on soft-tissue sarcomas below. Overall incidence and age distribution for rhabdoid renal tumour, CCSK and renal carcinoma were similar to those observed in Europe as a whole (Pastore *et al.*, 2006b). In a series of over 100 rhabdoid renal tumours from the NWTS, the median age at diagnosis was just below 1 year and there was an excess of boys (Weeks *et al.*, 1989).

3.9 Hepatic tumours

Hepatoblastoma is the rarest of the principal distinctive embryonal tumours of childhood. The ASR was 1.2 per million, representing 0.8% of all childhood cancers. Incidence was highest in the first 2 years of life, declining steeply thereafter (Fig. 3.21). There was a marked excess of boys, and the sex ratio varied little with age (Fig. 3.27). Hepatic carcinoma was rare throughout childhood. The incidence increased with age, with the majority of cases diagnosed at age 10–14 years; the youngest case in this series was diagnosed at 1 year of age. Boys and girls were affected equally. All of

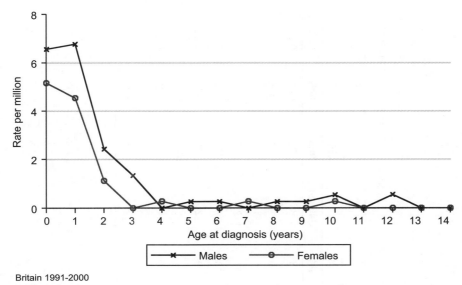

Britain 1991-2000

Fig. 3.27 Annual incidence rates by single year of age for hepatoblastoma, by sex, Great Britain, 1991–2000.

the registered cases were hepatocellular carcinoma (HCC) and there were no cases of cholangiocarcinoma. Fibrolamellar carcinoma accounted for 36% and other HCC for the remaining 64%.

In addition to hepatoblastoma and HCC, other types of childhood cancer can occur with the liver as primary site (Table 3.20). Inclusion of these tumours increases the total incidence of liver cancer in childhood by about a quarter, and this should be borne in mind when comparing incidence rates classified according to ICCC with those based purely on site. The most frequent of the other types of liver tumour were sarcomas, which in this series had an incidence only slightly below that of HCC. Lymphomas, neuroblastoma and germ cell tumours were also seen.

The incidence of hepatoblastoma and HCC was typical of that in European countries (Stiller *et al.*, 2006d). A somewhat higher incidence of hepatoblastoma has been found in North America, Israel and, especially, Japan (Parkin *et al.*, 1998; Bulterys *et al.*, 1999). In at least some of those countries, the excess compared to Europe was most pronounced among infants.

Hardly any population-based data have been published on childhood liver tumours other than hepatoblastoma and HCC. Among 42 children diagnosed in the West Midlands region of England during 1957–86, sarcomas accounted for 21% of the total and germ cell tumours for 7% (Mann *et al.*, 1990).

3.10 **Malignant bone tumours**

Incidence of malignant bone tumours increased with age (Fig. 3.28). The two sexes had similar incidence rates. The two most frequent subgroups of malignant bone tumours

Table 3.20 Numbers of registrations and age-standardized annual incidence per million children for malignant liver tumours, Great Britain, 1991–2000

Age group (years) at diagnosis	Registrations				Total			ASR		
	0	1–4	5–9	10–14	Boys	Girls	Children	Boys	Girls	Children
	Children									
Lymphoma	1	3	2	2	5	3	8	0.09	0.06	0.08
Neuroblastoma and ganglioneuroblastoma	0	1	0	0	1	0	1	0.02	0.00	0.01
Hepatoblastoma	42	60	5	5	71	41	112	1.45	0.89	1.18
Hepatic carcinoma	0	3	7	15	12	13	25	0.21	0.22	0.22
Sarcoma	9	6	5	2	13	9	22	0.26	0.19	0.22
Germ cell tumours	2	3	0	0	3	2	5	0.06	0.04	0.05
Unspecified malignant hepatic tumours	0	1	0	0	1	0	1	0.02	0.00	0.01
Total	54	77	19	24	106	68	174	2.11	1.41	1.77

ASR, age-standardized rate based on World Standard Population

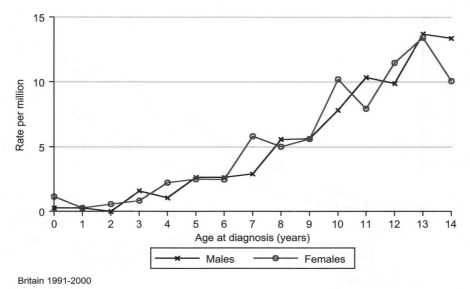

Britain 1991-2000

Fig. 3.28 Annual incidence rates by single year of age for malignant bone tumours, by sex, Great Britain, 1991–2000.

among children were osteosarcomas and Ewing tumour and related bone sarcomas (principally pPNET of bone). Osteosarcoma occurred more often, accounting for 55% of bone tumours and 2.1% of all childhood cancers. More than two-thirds of cases of osteosarcoma were diagnosed at age 10–14 years and only 1.6% at 1–4 years (Fig. 3.29); there were no registrations for children aged under 3 years. Slightly more girls than boys were affected in all age groups. Osteosarcoma in children is overwhelmingly a tumour of the long bones of the limbs. In this series, 84% of known primary sites were in the legs and 12% in the arms (Table 3.21). There was little variation in age or sex by primary site.

Ewing tumour of bone had a lower incidence than osteosarcoma. The majority of cases were again in children aged 10–14 years, but the predominance of older children was not quite as pronounced as for osteosarcoma. Indeed, up to the age of 6 years this subgroup was the most frequent type of malignant bone tumour (Fig. 3.29). Ewing tumour occurred equally frequently among boys and girls at ages 0–4 and 5–9 years, but at age 10–14 years there was a male excess (M:F = 1.2:1). The most common primary site was the long bones of the leg, 38% of cases of known site (Table 3.21). Substantial numbers of cases also arose in the pelvis (23%), long bones of the arm (11%), ribs, sternum and clavicle (9%) and spinal column (8%). Ewing tumour was by far the most frequent malignant tumour of the pelvis (78%) and ribs, sternum and clavicle (80%).

By comparison with osteosarcoma and Ewing tumour, other malignant bone tumours were very rare. The most frequent was chondrosarcoma but even for this tumour there

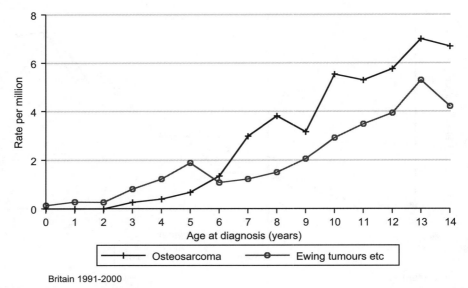

Britain 1991-2000

Fig. 3.29 Annual incidence rates by single year of age for osteosarcoma and Ewing's sarcoma of bone, Great Britain, 1991–2000.

was an average of only slightly more than 1 case per year in children throughout Great Britain. Nine of the 16 children in the subgroup of other specified malignant bone tumours had chordoma; they were predominantly 10–14 years of age at diagnosis and all but one were girls. The remaining 7 tumours comprised a wide range of different rare histological types.

Osteosarcoma had a similar incidence rate to those in most European countries (Stiller *et al.*, 2006a). It appears to be slightly more common in the United States (Gurney *et al.*, 1999c).

The incidence of Ewing tumour was low compared to many other series (Gurney *et al.*, 1999c; Desandes *et al.*, 2004; Stiller *et al.*, 2006a), but this may in part be due to varying allocation of tumours to bone and extraskeletal sites. Patterns of incidence for the Ewing sarcoma family of tumours in all sites combined are discussed after the section on soft tissue sarcomas below.

While the incidence of osteosarcoma in childhood is similar in boys and girls, a pronounced male excess starts at around the age of 15–16 years (dos Santos Silva and Swerdlow, 1993; Gurney *et al.*, 1999c; Stiller *et al.*, 2006a). Sex differences in bone sarcoma incidence in adolescents have been linked to parallel differences in skeletal growth between males and females (dos Santos Silva and Swerdlow, 1993), but there has been no suggested reason for the earlier emergence of the male excess in Ewing tumour compared with osteosarcoma. Chondrosarcoma and other types of malignant bone tumour are rare among children, as found in other reported series (Gurney *et al.*, 1999c; Stiller *et al.*, 2006a).

Table 3.21 Numbers of registrations for malignant bone tumours by histological type and primary site, Great Britain, 1991–2000

Histological type	Primary site											Total
	Long bones of arm	Hand and wrist	Long bones of leg	Foot and ankle	Skull and jaw	Spine	Rib, sternum and clavicle	Pelvic	Brain	Spinal cord	Unspecified	
Lymphoma	4	0	5	0	1	2	3	2	0	0	4	21
Osteosarcoma	37	0	254	0	1	2	1	8	0	0	4	307
Chondrosarcoma	3	1	3	1	2	1	1	0	0	0	0	12
Ewing/pPNET	24	1	83	11	9	18	20	50	0	0	1	217
Chordoma	0	0	0	0	2	3	0	1	2	1	0	9
Other specified bone tumours	0	0	4	0	1	1	0	1	0	0	0	7
Soft-tissue sarcoma	1	0	2	0	2	0	0	0	0	0	0	5
Unspecified	2	0	3	0	2	0	0	2	0	0	2	11
Total	71	2	354	12	20	27	25	64	2	1	11	589

3.11 **Soft tissue and other extraosseous sarcomas**

Collectively, the histologically diverse group of soft tissue and other extraosseous sarcomas accounted for 7% of all childhood cancers. Incidence of all these sarcomas combined was highest in infancy (Fig. 3.30). There was a sizeable male excess at ages between 3 and 8 years, but at both lower and higher ages the incidence was similar among boys and girls.

The predominant subgroup was rhabdomyosarcoma, accounting for 53% of soft tissue sarcomas and 3.7% of all cancers. The highest incidence of rhabdomyosarcoma was around 3 years of age (Fig. 3.31). Boys were affected 45% more often than girls. As with soft tissue sarcomas overall, however, the male excess was concentrated in the age range 3–8 years. Embryonal rhabdomyosarcoma was the predominant histological subtype, accounting for 62% of registrations (Table 3.22). Alveolar rhabdomyosarcoma (22%) was the only other subtype to occur in substantial numbers; 13% were of unspecified subtype and only 2% of other specified subtypes. Embryonal tumours tended to be registered in slightly younger children though all subtypes were represented in all age groups. The sex ratio was similar for embryonal and alveolar rhabdomyosarcoma.

Rhabdomyosarcoma can occur in almost all parts of the body. Table 3.23 shows the distribution by topographical grouping. Head and neck sites accounted for 41% of the total, genitourinary sites for 24%, other and unspecified sites in the trunk for 23%, and limbs for 10%. Histological subtype varied by site. Embryonal rhabdomyosarcoma predominated in all site groupings except the limbs, accounting for 65% of head and neck, 79% of genitourinary and 60% of other trunk. Alveolar rhabdomyosarcoma, however, was the most frequent subtype for limb primaries (54%).

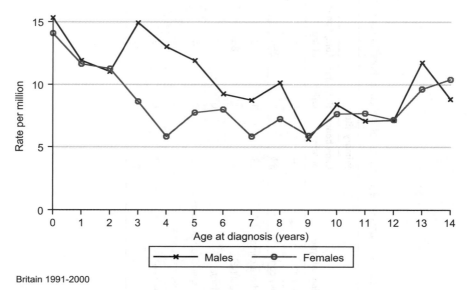

Britain 1991-2000

Fig. 3.30 Annual incidence rates by single year of age for soft tissue and other extraosseous sarcomas, by sex, Great Britain, 1991–2000.

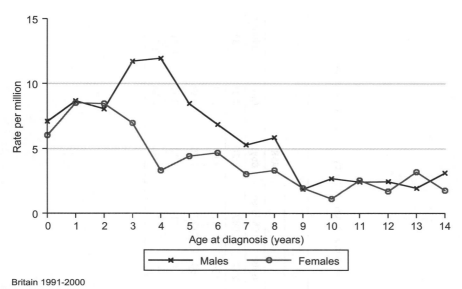

Britain 1991-2000

Fig. 3.31 Annual incidence rates by single year of age for rhabdomyosarcoma, by sex, Great Britain, 1991–2000.

Fibrosarcoma, malignant peripheral nerve sheath tumours (MPNSTs) and other fibrous neoplasms accounted for less than a tenth of soft tissue and other extraosseous sarcomas. Patterns of occurrence varied strikingly between the different divisions of this subgroup (Table 3.24). Incidence of fibroblastic and myofibroblastic tumours, predominantly fibrosarcoma, was similar among males and females. Incidence was highest in the first year of life, then fell sharply before increasing again through the remainder of childhood. Twelve of the 13 tumours in infants, and 4 in older children, were specified as infantile fibrosarcoma. MPNST were predominantly tumours of older children, and there was a marked excess of girls (sex ratio 0.6:1).

Kaposi sarcoma was exceedingly rare, with only five registrations during the ten-year period.

Other specified soft tissue sarcomas formed the second largest subgroup after rhabdomyosarcoma (Table 3.25). Peripheral primitive neuroectodermal tumours (pPNETs), together with Ewing and Askin tumours of soft tissue, accounted for 44% of the total. Their incidence was fairly constant in the first 10 years of life, and increased slightly thereafter. These tumours occurred mainly in the trunk (62%), with 36% specified as thoracic. There were no cases in genitourinary sites other than the kidney; pPNET of this site are classified with the diagnostic group of renal tumours. The remaining pPNET were evenly divided between the head and neck and the limbs.

The other principal types in this subgroup were synovial sarcoma (17%), fibrohistiocytic tumours (14%), extrarenal rhabdoid tumour (6%) and leiomyosarcoma (4%).

Text starts on page 88

Table 3.22 Numbers of registrations and age-standardized annual incidence per million children for rhabdomyosarcoma by histological subtype, Great Britain, 1991–2000

Age group (years) at diagnosis	Registrations				Total			ASR		
	0	1–4	5–9	10–14	Boys	Girls	Children	Boys	Girls	Children
	Children									
Total	**47**	**248**	**170**	**82**	**330**	**217**	**547**	**6.26**	**4.31**	**5.31**
Embryonal	29	165	112	35	206	135	341	3.94	2.71	3.34
Alveolar	11	46	37	29	73	50	123	1.36	0.97	1.17
Other specified	1	5	2	3	6	5	11	0.12	0.10	0.11
Unspecified	6	32	19	15	45	27	72	0.84	0.54	0.69

ASR, age-standardized rate based on World Standard Population

Table 3.23 Numbers of registrations for rhabdomyosarcoma by histological subtype and primary site, Great Britain, 1991–2000

| Histological subtype | Primary site | | | | | | | |
	Orbit	Other head and neck	Bladder, prostate	Other genito-urinary	Other trunk	Extremity	Unspecified	Total
Embryonal	35	113	51	51	75	14	2	341
Alveolar	8	36	1	10	32	29	7	123
Other	1	3	0	2	2	3	0	11
Unspecified	7	23	2	12	17	8	3	72
Total	51	175	54	75	126	54	12	547

Table 3.24 Numbers of registrations and age-standardized annual incidence per million children for fibrosarcomas, peripheral nerve sheath tumours and other fibrous neoplasms, Great Britain, 1991–2000

Age group (years) at diagnosis	Registrations				Total			ASR		
	0	1–4	5–9	10–14	Boys	Girls	Children	Boys	Girls	Children
	Children									
Total	**16**	**9**	**18**	**37**	**34**	**46**	**80**	**0.62**	**0.85**	**0.73**
Fibroblastic and myofibroblastic tumours	13	5	6	13	19	18	37	0.36	0.35	0.35
Nerve sheath tumours	3	4	10	24	15	26	41	0.26	0.47	0.36
Other fibromatous neoplasms	0	0	2	0	0	2	2	0.00	0.04	0.02

ASR, age-standardized rate based on World Standard Population

Table 3.25 Numbers of registrations and age-standardized annual incidence per million children for other specified soft tissue sarcomas, Great Britain, 1991–2000

Age group (years) at diagnosis	Registrations				Total			ASR		
	0	1–4	5–9	10–14	Boys	Girls	Children	Boys	Girls	Children
	Children									
Total	**32**	**58**	**91**	**159**	**179**	**161**	**340**	**3.16**	**2.97**	**3.07**
Ewing tumour and Askin tumour of soft tissue	0	4	10	15	15	14	29	0.26	0.25	0.25
Peripheral neuroectodermal tumour (pPNET) of soft tissue	10	31	34	47	57	65	122	1.03	1.22	1.12
Extrarenal rhabdoid tumour	12	3	2	2	6	13	19	0.13	0.27	0.20
Liposarcomas	1	0	0	3	2	2	4	0.04	0.03	0.04
Fibrohistiocytic tumours	4	3	14	26	29	18	47	0.51	0.31	0.41
Malignant fibrous histiocytoma	1	2	5	14	12	10	22	0.21	0.17	0.19
Dermatofibrosarcoma protuberans	3	1	9	11	16	8	24	0.28	0.14	0.21
Malignant giant cell tumour	0	0	0	1	1	0	1	0.02	0.00	0.01
Leiomyosarcomas	0	1	4	7	6	6	12	0.10	0.10	0.10
Synovial sarcomas	0	4	13	41	38	20	58	0.62	0.36	0.49
Blood vessel tumours	2	5	0	4	6	5	11	0.11	0.10	0.11
Osseous and chondromatous	1	0	4	4	4	5	9	0.07	0.09	0.08
Alveolar soft part sarcoma	0	1	5	4	3	7	10	0.05	0.13	0.09
Miscellaneous soft tissue sarcomas	2	6	5	6	13	6	19	0.24	0.12	0.18

ASR, age-standardized rate based on World Standard Population

Synovial sarcoma occurred mostly in older children, and the majority (31/58, 53%) had their primary site in the lower limbs. Fibrohistiocytic tumours were evenly divided between malignant fibrous histiocytoma (MFH) and dermatofibrosarcoma protuberans (DFSP). Incidence of MFH increased with age and there was a small male excess. DFSP was most frequent at age 10–14 years but there was also a peak in infancy; boys were affected twice as often as girls. Extrarenal rhabdoid tumour, like rhabdoid renal tumour, had its highest incidence among infants. The predominance of girls, however, was in marked contrast to the male excess in rhabdoid renal tumour. The 11 blood vessel tumours comprised 6 angiosarcomas and 5 malignant haemangioendotheliomas; they were most frequent in the first 5 years of life. All but one of the osseous and chondromatous neoplasms of soft tissue were chondrosarcomas. Alveolar soft part sarcoma was remarkable for the predominance of girls. The 19 miscellaneous soft tissue sarcomas comprised 12 cases of desmoplastic small round cell tumour (DSRCT), 3 each of mesenchymoma and ectomesenchymoma and a single myxosarcoma.

Finally, unspecified soft tissue sarcomas accounted for 6% of the total. They were most frequent in infancy and at age 10–14. These tumours occurred with similar frequency among boys and girls.

Incidence rates for all soft tissue sarcomas combined and for rhabdomyosarcoma were similar to the European average (Pastore *et al.*, 2006a). In the United States, the ratio of incidence rates for embryonal to alveolar rhabdomyosarcoma was 4.3:1 (Gurney *et al.*, 1999e), rather higher than the 2.9:1 in Britain. The American data, however, related to the period 1975–95, on average 10 years before the present study, and an increase in the proportion of cases classified as alveolar would be expected following the adoption of cytological criteria for diagnosis (Asmar *et al.*, 1994). The divergent age-incidence pattern between boys and girls for rhabdomyosarcoma does not seem to have been reported previously. The American rates for fibrosarcoma, MFH and DFSP (Gurney *et al.*, 1999e) were all 1.5–3 times those in Britain. The American data covered an earlier period and, at least for fibrosarcoma and MFH, the differences may simply reflect a marked decrease in the frequency with which tumours are assigned to these categories by pathologists (Daugaard, 2004). The very low incidence of Kaposi sarcoma in childhood is typical of industrialized countries with a relatively low frequency of vertically transmitted HIV infection (Mueller, 1999). Britain and the United States had similar incidence rates for MPNST and synovial sarcoma, but extraosseous Ewing tumour and pPNET had an incidence of only 0.3 per million in the United States (Gurney *et al.*, 1999e), less than one-quarter of the rate in Britain.

3.12 Overview of Ewing sarcoma family of tumours and rhabdoid tumours

Total age-standardized incidence of the Ewing sarcoma family of tumours (ESFTs) was 3.3 per million (Table 3.26), and they accounted for 2.4% of total childhood cancer incidence. Boys and girls were affected equally and 55% of cases were diagnosed at age 10–14 years. The primary site was bone in 58% of cases. Bone primaries tended to occur

Table 3.26 Numbers of registrations and age-standardized annual incidence per million children for Ewing sarcoma family of tumours (ESFTs), Great Britain, 1991–2000

Age group (years) at diagnosis	Registrations				Total			ASR		
	Children	1–4	5–9	10–14	Boys	Girls	Children	Boys	Girls	Children
	0									
Total	**12**	**54**	**104**	**205**	**192**	**183**	**375**	**3.30**	**3.30**	**3.30**
Ewing tumour of bone and related bone sarcomas	1	19	57	140	117	100	217	1.95	1.76	1.86
Ewing tumour and Askin tumour of soft tissue	0	4	10	15	15	14	29	0.26	0.25	0.25
Peripheral neuroectodermal tumour (pPNET) of soft tissue	10	31	34	47	57	65	122	1.03	1.22	1.12
Peripheral neuroectodermal tumour (pPNET) of kidney	1	0	3	3	3	4	7	0.05	0.07	0.06

ASR, age-standardized rate based on World Standard Population

in older children than extraosseous tumours; the ratio of bone to non-bone sites increased from 0.1:1 at age 0 to 0.5:1 at age 1–4, 1.2:1 at age 5–9 and 2.2:1 at age 10–14.

While it has been recognized for a while that it makes sense epidemiologically to consider all ESFT together (Valery *et al.*, 2002), we believe this is the first time that incidence rates have been presented for the group as a whole. As remarked in the discussion of bone tumours above, the incidence rate for Ewing tumour of bone was lower than in many other series (Gurney *et al.*, 1999c; Desandes *et al.*, 2004; Stiller *et al.*, 2006a). The total incidence of ESFT in Britain, however, exceeded that reported for Ewing tumour of bone in most other countries, and it seems likely that this is partly due to a greater readiness to record tumours of the ESFT as having an extraosseous site in more recent years.

Rhabdoid tumours of all sites combined had an age-standardized incidence of 0.7 per million (Table 3.27). Regardless of site, these were predominantly neoplasms of very young children. Boys and girls had similar incidence rates for all sites combined and for ATRT, but there was a pronounced male excess for rhabdoid renal tumour, counterbalanced by a female excess of similar magnitude for other extrarenal sites.

3.13 **Germ cell tumours, trophoblastic tumours and neoplasms of gonads**

This group as a whole accounted for 3.3% of all registrations. Within the group, 98% were germ cell tumours and only 2% were carcinomas. The distributions of germ cell tumours by age and sex varied markedly with primary site. Intracranial and intraspinal tumours accounted for 35% of all germ cell tumours. The incidence was highest at age 10–14 years and they were slightly more common among boys than girls overall (Fig. 3.32). Among children aged under 5 years girls were affected more often than boys, whereas at older ages there was a male excess, with the sex ratio reaching 1.9:1 by age 10–14 years. The most frequent histological subtypes were germinomas (53%) and teratomas (35%) (Table 3.28). Non-malignant tumours accounted for 57% of the teratomas and for 20% of all intracranial and intraspinal germ cell tumours. Incidence of germinomas increased with age, whereas teratomas had a peak in infancy and lower, but fairly constant, incidence thereafter.

Other extragonadal sites accounted for 22% of germ cell tumours. These tumours occurred almost entirely before age 5 years and they were twice as frequent among girls as among boys. Half of them were yolk sac tumours and 41% were teratomas (Table 3.29); the female excess was especially prominent for yolk sac tumours. Pelvic sites accounted for 55% of the subgroup, abdominal and retroperitoneal for 20% and mediastinal and other thoracic for 15% (Table 3.30). The female excess was most marked for pelvic sites, even after the exclusion of those in the female reproductive tract. The majority of thoracic tumours were in boys. All sites were most frequently affected in early childhood, but one-third of the tumours in children aged 5–14 years were thoracic.

Malignant gonadal germ cell tumours had strikingly different age distributions in the two sexes (Fig. 3.33). In boys, testicular tumours had their peak incidence in the second

Table 3.27 Numbers of registrations and age-standardized annual incidence per million children for rhabdoid tumours, Great Britain, 1991–2000

Age group (years) at diagnosis	Registrations				Total			ASR		
	0	1–4	5–9	10–14	Boys	Girls	Children	Boys	Girls	Children
	Children									
Total	**34**	**23**	**5**	**5**	**35**	**32**	**67**	**0.72**	**0.68**	**0.70**
Atypical teratoid/rhabdoid tumour of CNS	8	10	3	3	12	12	24	0.23	0.25	0.24
Rhabdoid renal tumour	14	10	0	0	17	7	24	0.36	0.15	0.26
Extrarenal rhabdoid tumour	12	3	2	2	6	13	19	0.13	0.27	0.20

ASR, age-standardized rate based on World Standard Population

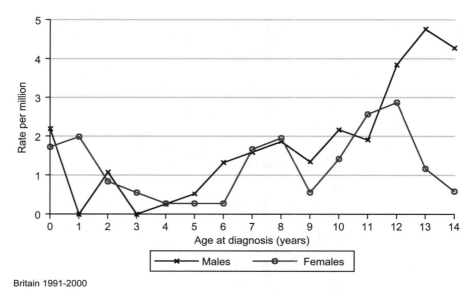

Britain 1991-2000

Fig. 3.32 Annual incidence rates by single year of age for intracranial and intraspinal germ cell tumours, by sex, Great Britain, 1991–2000.

year of life, and they were almost never seen at age 3–12 years, but incidence increased again at age 13–14 years. In young boys they were nearly always yolk sac tumours whereas at age 10–14 they were predominantly malignant teratomas and seminomas (Table 3.31). In girls, by contrast, the incidence of ovarian germ cell tumours increased with age throughout childhood. There were no registrations at all in the first year of life and very few at age 1–4 years. Two-thirds of cases occurred at age 10–14. Teratomas accounted for 47%, dysgerminomas for 23% and yolk sac tumours for 19%.

Gonadal carcinomas were very rare and were nearly always in the ovaries of girls aged 5–14 years; the one case in a boy was of testicular carcinoid. There were only two cases in the subgroup of other and unspecified gonadal tumours; both were unspecified testicular tumours in boys.

Incidence of germ cell tumours relative to other countries varied according to primary site. The rates for intracranial and intraspinal tumours were similar to those in several European countries (Parkin *et al.*, 1988a, 1998; Stiller and Parkin, 1996; Kaatsch *et al.*, 2001; Desandes *et al.*, 2004), though some, including the Netherlands (Netherlands Cancer Registry, 2000), had higher incidence while others, especially those which excluded non-malignant tumours, had lower rates. In the United States, the incidence rates from the SEER registries for 1990–95 were similar to those in Britain despite being based only on malignant tumours (Bernstein *et al.*, 1999b). The incidence rate in the CBTRUS, however, which includes non-malignant tumours, was also very similar to that in the present study (CBTRUS, 2002). For other extragonadal sites, incidence in Britain was similar to the European average, but the United States had slightly higher incidence, 1.1 per million in boys and 1.9 per million in girls in 1990–95 (Bernstein *et al.*, 1999b).

Text starts on page 96

Table 3.28 Numbers of registrations and age-standardized annual incidence per million children for intracranial and intraspinal germ cell tumours by ICCC-3 division (histological subtype), Great Britain, 1991–2000

Age group (years) at diagnosis	Registrations (Children)				Total			ASR		
	0	1–4	5–9	10–14	Boys	Girls	Children	Boys	Girls	Children
Total	**14**	**18**	**42**	**91**	**99**	**66**	**165**	**1.68**	**1.22**	**1.46**
Intracranial and intraspinal germinomas	1	2	17	67	49	38	87	0.80	0.66	0.73
Intracranial and intraspinal teratomas	13	13	18	14	34	24	58	0.61	0.49	0.55
Intracranial and intraspinal embryonal carcinomas	0	0	2	2	3	1	4	0.05	0.02	0.03
Intracranial and intraspinal yolk sac tumour	0	3	1	2	5	1	6	0.09	0.02	0.06
Intracranial and intraspinal choriocarcinoma	0	0	1	0	1	0	1	0.02	0.00	0.01
Intracranial and intraspinal tumours of mixed forms	0	0	3	6	7	2	9	0.11	0.04	0.08

ASR, age-standardized rate based on World Standard Population

Table 3.29 Numbers of registrations and age-standardized annual incidence per million children for malignant extracranial and extragonadal germ cell tumours by ICCC-3 division (histological subtype), Great Britain, 1991–2000

Age group (years) at diagnosis	Registrations				Total			ASR		
	Children				Boys	Girls	Children	Boys	Girls	Children
	0	1–4	5–9	10–14						
Total	43	52	4	8	34	73	107	0.70	1.57	1.12
Malignant germinomas of extracranial and extragonadal sites	0	1	0	1	1	1	2	0.02	0.02	0.02
Malignant teratomas of extracranial and extragonadal sites	31	8	2	3	20	24	44	0.41	0.52	0.46
Embryonal carcinomas of extracranial and extragonadal sites	0	0	1	0	0	1	1	0.00	0.02	0.01
Yolk sac tumour of extracranial and extragonadal sites	10	41	1	2	10	44	54	0.21	0.95	0.57
Choriocarcinomas of extracranial and extragonadal sites	2	0	0	1	2	1	3	0.04	0.02	0.03
Other and unspecified malignant mixed germ cell tumours of extracranial and extragonadal sites	0	2	0	1	1	2	3	0.02	0.04	0.03

ASR, age-standardized rate based on World Standard Population

Table 3.30 Numbers of registrations and age-standardized annual incidence per million children for malignant extracranial and extragonadal germ cell tumours by primary site, Great Britain, 1991–2000

Age group (years) at diagnosis	Registrations					Total			ASR		
	Children	0	1–4	5–9	10–14	Boys	Girls	Children	Boys	Girls	Children
Total	**43**	**52**	**4**	**8**		**34**	**73**	**107**	**0.70**	**1.56**	**1.12**
Head and neck	4	1	0	1		3	3	6	0.06	0.07	0.06
Thoracic	4	8	1	3		10	6	16	0.20	0.12	0.16
Liver	2	3	0	0		3	2	5	0.06	0.04	0.05
Other abdominal	9	7	0	0		8	8	16	0.17	0.18	0.17
Female reproductive	4	6	1	1		0	12	12	0.00	0.25	0.12
Other pelvic	17	26	2	2		7	40	47	0.14	0.86	0.49
Unspecified	3	1	0	1		3	2	5	0.06	0.04	0.05

ASR, age-standardized rate based on World Standard Population

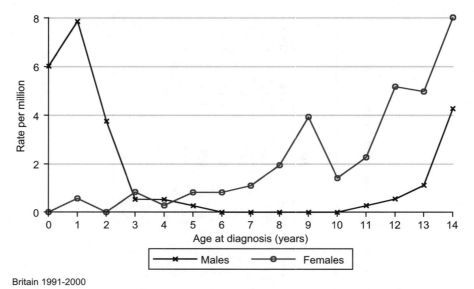

Britain 1991-2000

Fig. 3.33 Annual incidence rates by single year of age for malignant gonadal germ cell tumours, by sex, Great Britain, 1991–2000.

Incidence of gonadal germ cell tumours was also typical of that in European countries. In the United States, the incidence of testicular germ cell tumours was similar to that in Britain, whereas the incidence of ovarian germ cell tumours was about 50% higher (Bernstein *et al.*, 1999b). The age distributions for all combinations of site and sex were broadly similar to those observed elsewhere. The upturn in testicular germ cell tumours around 12–13 years of age marks the start of a steep rise in incidence with age, such that among adolescent and young adult males aged 15–24 years testicular cancer is one of the most common malignancies in many populations (Smith *et al.*, 1999b). The incidence of ovarian carcinoma was appreciably lower than it had been in Britain and several other countries during the 1980s (Parkin *et al.*, 1998), or in the SEER registries during 1990–95 (Bernstein *et al.*, 1999b). This is undoubtedly an artefact resulting from the upgrading of certain borderline tumours to malignant in the second edition of ICD-O (Bernstein *et al.*, 1999b), and their consequent inclusion in ICCC (Kramárová and Stiller, 1996), followed by their downgrading to uncertain behaviour in the third edition and exclusion from ICCC-3 (Steliarova-Foucher *et al.*, 2005b). During 1991–2000 in Britain, there were seven registrations for these borderline tumours, the same number as for the ovarian carcinomas that appear in Table 3.1.

3.14 Other malignant epithelial neoplasms and malignant melanomas

This group includes carcinomas of all sites except kidney, liver and gonads, together with malignant melanoma. The group as a whole accounted for 3.3% of all childhood

Table 3.31 Numbers of registrations and age-standardized annual incidence per million children for malignant gonadal germ cell tumours by ICCC-3 division (histological subtype), Great Britain, 1991–2000

Age group (years) at diagnosis	Registrations				Total			ASR		
	Children				Boys	Girls	Children	Boys	Girls	Children
	0	1–4	5–9	10–14						
Total	22	53	32	97	92	112	204	1.81	1.95	1.88
Malignant gonadal germinomas	0	2	8	22	6	26	32	0.10	0.45	0.27
Malignant gonadal teratomas	6	3	18	48	22	53	75	0.39	0.92	0.65
Gonadal embryonal carcinomas	0	0	0	1	0	1	1	0.00	0.02	0.01
Gonadal yolk sac tumour	16	46	3	17	61	21	82	1.27	0.36	0.83
Gonadal choriocarcinoma	0	0	0	1	0	1	1	0.00	0.02	0.01
Malignant gonadal tumours of mixed forms	0	2	3	8	3	10	13	0.05	0.18	0.11

ASR, age-standardized rate based on World Standard Population

cancers, while carcinomas, including those of the kidney, liver and gonads, accounted for 2.6%. Most carcinomas and melanomas are characteristically cancers of adulthood and, even within childhood, the incidence increases steeply with age; two-thirds of registrations in this group were for children aged 10–14 years. Girls were affected somewhat more often than boys.

Adrenocortical carcinoma (ACC) had an ASR of only 0.2 per million. Uniquely among childhood carcinomas, incidence was higher at age 1–4 years than among older children. ACC had twice the incidence in girls compared with boys.

The thyroid is one of the most frequent sites for carcinomas in children. Thyroid carcinoma accounted for 19% of all carcinomas including those in other diagnostic groups. Incidence increased with age. Only 7% of registrations were for children diagnosed before age 5 years, and 69% of cases were in the 10–14 year age group. Thyroid carcinoma was about twice as frequent among girls as among boys overall. Differentiated carcinoma (papillary or follicular) accounted for 63% of cases and medullary carcinoma for 37% (Table 3.32). Incidence of both subtypes increased with age. Medullary carcinoma, however, tended to be diagnosed at an earlier age than differentiated tumours, and nearly all the thyroid carcinomas diagnosed in the first 5 years of life were medullary. Differentiated carcinoma was more than twice as frequent among girls compared with boys (sex ratio 0.4:1), whereas medullary carcinoma occurred equally in the two sexes. Consequently, differentiated and medullary tumours were equally frequent among boys, whereas girls had a pronounced excess of differentiated carcinoma.

The incidence of nasopharyngeal carcinoma was about one-third that of thyroid carcinomas. This tumour was hardly ever seen in children below 10 years of age, and the youngest patient in this series was aged 6 years at diagnosis. Boys had an incidence rate more than four times that for girls. Undifferentiated or anaplastic carcinoma accounted for 42% of cases, squamous carcinoma for 25% and lymphoepithelial carcinoma for 8%; the remaining 25% were of unspecified histological subtype.

Malignant melanoma accounted for just over 1% of all childhood cancers. The incidence increased with age; 58% of registrations were for children aged 10 years and above. Girls were affected more frequently than boys (sex ratio 0.7:1). The great majority of malignant melanomas were cutaneous in origin (89%), but there were also primaries in the eye (5%) and central nervous system (6%) (Table 3.33). While there was a female excess of cutaneous melanoma, boys accounted for the majority of melanomas of the eye (6/8) and CNS (5/9). Boys and girls had similar numbers of cutaneous melanoma of the head and neck, but there was a female excess of melanomas of other skin sites (sex ratio 0.6:1). More than one-half of children with melanoma of the head and neck and of the CNS were aged under 10 years at diagnosis, whereas melanomas of other skin sites and of the eye were predominantly diagnosed at 10–14 years of age.

The recorded incidence of skin carcinomas was slightly more than half that of malignant melanoma. Two-thirds of registrations were for children aged 10–14 years. There was a small male excess. The two main histological subtypes were squamous cell carcinoma and basal cell carcinoma (BCC), accounting respectively for 11 and 80% of registrations. The head and neck was the most frequent site for skin carcinomas,

Table 3.32 Numbers of registrations and age-standardized annual incidence per million children for thyroid carcinoma by histological subtype, Great Britain, 1991–2000

Age group (years) at diagnosis	Registrations					Total			ASR		
	0	1–4	5–9	10–14		Boys	Girls	Children	Boys	Girls	Children
	Children										
Total	**0**	**5**	**17**	**49**		**25**	**46**	**71**	**0.42**	**0.79**	**0.60**
Differentiated	0	1	12	32		13	32	45	0.21	0.55	0.38
Medullary	0	4	5	17		12	14	26	0.21	0.24	0.23

ASR, age-standardized rate based on World Standard Population

Table 3.33 Numbers of registrations and age-standardized annual incidence per million children for malignant melanoma by primary site, Great Britain, 1991–2000

Age group (years) at diagnosis	Registrations				Total			ASR		
	0	1–4	5–9	10–14	Boys	Girls	Children	Boys	Girls	Children
	Children									
Total	**7**	**19**	**39**	**89**	**65**	**89**	**154**	**1.09**	**1.63**	**1.35**
Skin of head and neck	1	7	7	7	11	11	22	0.19	0.22	0.20
Skin of trunk	1	1	5	15	9	13	22	0.15	0.23	0.19
Skin of upper limbs	0	2	12	24	14	24	38	0.23	0.42	0.32
Skin of lower limbs	0	4	11	29	15	29	44	0.25	0.51	0.38
Other and unspecified skin	4	1	2	4	5	6	11	0.09	0.12	0.10
Eye	0	1	0	7	6	2	8	0.10	0.04	0.07
CNS	1	3	2	3	5	4	9	0.09	0.08	0.08

ASR, age-standardized rate based on World Standard Population

accounting for 64% of all cases, followed by the trunk (20%) and limbs (10%); primary site was unspecified in the remaining 6%.

Among the subgroup of other and unspecified carcinomas, the most common specified primary sites were the salivary glands, appendix, colon and rectum, lung and bladder (Table 3.34). Eighty percent of all registrations in the subgroup were for children aged 10–14 years, with little variation by site. Girls were affected slightly more often than boys. The salivary gland tumours were mostly mucoepidermoid carcinomas (43%) and acinar cell carcinomas (27%). Ten (91%) of the 11 colorectal carcinomas were in the colon and 1 in the rectum. The 15 cases of carcinomas in the appendix comprised 14 carcinoid tumours and one signet ring cell carcinoma. Of the 10 lung tumours, 8 were bronchial adenomas and 2 were mucoepidermoid carcinomas. The 6 bladder carcinomas were all of transitional cell type.

In common with other carcinomas, the incidence of ACC is highest in older adults but, uniquely, there is also an age peak in early childhood which is generally found in population-based series with substantial numbers of cases (Stiller, 1994b; Correa and Chen, 1995; Bernstein and Gurney, 1999; Stiller et al., 2006b).

Thyroid carcinoma was rather uncommon by comparison with some other European regions (Steliarova-Foucher et al., 2006b). Higher incidence rates have also been consistently recorded in North America (Bernstein and Gurney, 1999). It seems likely that these variations reflect differences in the intensity of diagnostic activity between countries, though varying levels of ascertainment of detected cases and differences in underlying risk cannot be ruled out (Steliarova-Foucher et al., 2006b). The proportion of medullary carcinoma was higher than in a slightly overlapping national series of children diagnosed during 1963–92 (Harach and Williams, 1995). Among the subset of that series whose histology could be reviewed, no cases were transferred from differentiated to medullary or vice versa, and an increase in the incidence of medullary carcinoma over time was attributed to the development of screening for familial cases (Harach and Williams, 1995). The marked female excess for differentiated carcinoma and similar incidence of medullary carcinoma in boys and girls were typical of the pattern for Europe as a whole (Steliarova-Foucher et al., 2006b).

Incidence of nasopharyngeal carcinoma was similar to that in other western countries (Parkin et al., 1998; Bernstein and Gurney, 1999; Stiller et al., 2006b).

By far the highest incidence of malignant melanoma at all ages, and in childhood, is found in Australia, as a consequence of excess sun exposure in a susceptible population (McWhirter and Dobson, 1995). The incidence in Britain was fairly typical of European countries (de Vries et al., 2006). The rates reported here should be treated with caution, however, because the distinction between malignant, in-situ and 'benign' melanomas can be difficult. In population-based series from New Zealand, Denmark, Sweden and Finland, the proportion of registered cases of childhood malignant melanoma reclassified as non-malignant on review ranged from 40 to 96% (Saksela and Rintala, 1968; Malec and Lagerlof, 1977; Partoft et al., 1989; Dockerty et al., 1997). In a study of childhood melanoma in the West of Scotland, pathological review of 13 of the 20 cases diagnosed during 1979–2002 was possible (Leman et al., 2005). Eight (62%) of the

Table 3.34 Numbers of registrations and age-standardized annual incidence per million children for other and unspecified carcinomas, Great Britain, 1991–2000

Age group (years) at diagnosis	Registrations				Total			ASR		
	0	1–4	5–9	10–14	Boys	Girls	Children	Boys	Girls	Children
Total	**0**	**4**	**21**	**103**	**58**	**70**	**128**	**0.95**	**1.20**	**1.07**
Carcinomas of salivary glands	0	0	9	21	11	19	30	0.18	0.33	0.25
Carcinomas of colon and rectum	0	0	1	10	6	5	11	0.10	0.09	0.09
Carcinomas of appendix	0	0	1	14	6	9	15	0.10	0.15	0.12
Carcinomas of lung	0	0	2	8	6	4	10	0.10	0.07	0.08
Carcinomas of thymus	0	0	0	4	4	0	4	0.06	0.00	0.03
Carcinomas of cervix uteri	0	0	0	1	0	1	1	0.00	0.02	0.01
Carcinomas of bladder	0	0	1	5	4	2	6	0.07	0.03	0.05
Carcinomas of other specified sites	0	1	5	33	17	22	39	0.28	0.37	0.33
Carcinomas of unspecified site	0	3	2	7	4	8	12	0.07	0.15	0.11

ASR, age-standardized rate based on World Standard Population

reviewed cases, 40% of the complete series, were reclassified as unusual naevi. Moreover, the default coding in ICD and ICD-O for melanoma not otherwise specified assumes that it is malignant; while this is reasonably satisfactory for melanoma in adults, who account for the great majority of cases, it is less appropriate for childhood tumours. With these points in mind, a particular effort was made to confirm the malignancy of melanomas in this series. The site distribution by sex in Australia showed some differences from that in Britain, with a male excess for head and neck and similar numbers of boys and girls for trunk and arm, though there was a marked excess of girls with melanoma of the leg (McWhirter and Dobson, 1995). The tendency for melanoma of the head and neck to occur in younger children was also observed in the United States SEER registries (Strouse *et al.*, 2005).

Skin carcinoma is rare among children in all western populations (Parkin *et al.*, 1998; Bernstein and Gurney, 1999; de Vries *et al.*, 2006). These tumours tend to be under-registered and the incidence rates should therefore be regarded as minimum estimates (de Vries *et al.*, 2006). Furthermore, since children with skin carcinomas are rarely referred to paediatric oncologists and the prognosis is excellent, general cancer registries are the main source of notification to the NRCT, and virtually the only one for regions without a local specialist children's tumour registry. Registration of skin carcinoma is known to be variable in Britain; in particular, the Thames Cancer Registry, which covered about 24% of the population of Britain during the study period, ceased to register BCC from 1992 (Goodwin *et al.*, 2004). Therefore, it seems likely that the incidence rates of BCC and total skin carcinoma for 1991–2000 in the NRCT are underestimated by around 22 and 18% respectively, and that BCC represents about 85% of all skin carcinomas in children.

The total recorded incidence of carcinomas of other sites is heavily influenced by the policy of individual registries regarding the coding of carcinoid tumours of the appendix (Stiller *et al.*, 2006b). In children, this is usually a low-grade neoplasm which is generally diagnosed incidentally (Parkes *et al.*, 1993). It is unclear how many of the 14 carcinoid tumours of the appendix or 15 of unspecified sites within the digestive tract in this study were actually malignant. The overall incidence of other carcinomas was typical of European countries (Stiller *et al.*, 2006b).

3.15 Other and unspecified malignant neoplasms

The miscellaneous subgroup of other specified malignant tumours accounted for only 0.1% of all childhood cancers. The histological types represented were pancreatoblastoma, pleuropulmonary blastoma, mesothelioma and gastrointestinal stromal tumour (Table 3.35). Of these, pleuropulmonary blastoma was the most numerous with eight registrations; as three of them were originally registered as sarcomas, it seems likely that the incidence of this rare tumour is underestimated. There were no cases of pulmonary blastoma, which is included in the same division of ICCC-3.

Finally, the somewhat larger subgroup of other unspecified malignant tumours contained tumours of sites other than the CNS, kidney, liver, bone and gonads, for

Table 3.35 Numbers of registrations and age-standardized annual incidence per million children for other specified malignant tumours, Great Britain, 1991–2000

Age group (years) at diagnosis	Registrations				Total			ASR		
	0	1–4	5–9	10–14	Boys	Girls	Children	Boys	Girls	Children
	Children									
Total	**2**	**8**	**1**	**6**	**8**	**9**	**17**	**0.15**	**0.18**	**0.16**
Gastrointestinal stromal tumour	1	0	0	1	1	1	2	0.02	0.02	0.02
Pancreatoblastoma	0	1	1	2	3	1	4	0.05	0.02	0.04
Pulmonary blastoma and pleuropulmonary blastoma	1	6	0	1	4	4	8	0.08	0.09	0.08
Mesothelioma	0	1	0	2	0	3	3	0.00	0.06	0.03

ASR, age-standardized rate based on World Standard Population

which there was little or no information available on histological type. These tumours were rather more frequent in the first year of life than subsequently.

3.16 Conclusions

The incidence of childhood cancer in Britain was broadly similar to that in other western countries. While the analysis of variations between the constituent countries of the UK or between smaller geographical areas within them is outside the scope of this volume, the incidence rates for Great Britain as a whole can be compared with those in the recent, comprehensive study of childhood cancer in Scotland (Campbell *et al.*, 2004). The Scottish results were generally similar to those for the whole of Britain. The main exception concerns CNS tumours, group III and subgroup Xa in ICCC-3, for which the rates in Scotland were somewhat lower. This is because, although non-malignant intracranial and intraspinal tumours are recorded by the Scottish Cancer Registry, the published incidence rates were for malignant tumours only.

The incidence data published here are the first in which the diagnoses are categorized according to ICCC-3. The newly created divisions of ICCC-3 were mostly applicable to these data from the 1990s, except for the uncertainties resulting from terminological ambiguities in NHL. We hope that these results will be a suitable basis of comparison for other population-based data on childhood cancer incidence using ICCC-3.

Chapter 4

Time Trends in Incidence 1966–2000

ME Kroll and CA Stiller

4.1 Introduction

This chapter contains a descriptive analysis of time trends in the incidence of childhood cancer in Great Britain from 1966 to 2000. Results are presented for all cancers together, and for diagnostic groups and subgroups of the third edition of the International Classification of Childhood Cancers (ICCC-3), by age group or sex wherever appropriate. A major problem in the interpretation of the data is that diagnostic methods and terminology have changed over time. Possible consequences are discussed, including the extent to which (usually increasing) trends for very specific diagnostic categories reflect changes in the opposite direction for less specific categories, and the extent and timing of shifts or exchanges between diagnostic groups.

Table 4.1 presents the total numbers of cases diagnosed during 1966–2000 and the age-standardized rate in each successive five-year period, for diagnostic groups and subgroups and for all cancers combined. Cases from diagnostic groups that were not part of the second edition of ICCC (ICCC-2) were excluded because of probable incomplete ascertainment in the earlier years. The effect, with the exclusions described in Chapter 4, is to simplify slightly the leukaemia classification: 'leukaemias, myeloproliferative and myelodysplastic diseases' is reduced to 'leukaemias', 'chronic myeloproliferative diseases' becomes 'chronic myeloid leukaemia' (CML) and 'myelodysplastic syndrome and other myeloproliferative diseases' becomes 'juvenile/chronic myelomonocytic leukaemias' (JMML/CMML).

Figures 4.1–4.4 illustrate changes over time in recorded rates of leukaemias, lymphomas, CNS tumours and a selection of solid tumours, based on a simplified ICCC-3 classification.

The time trend in each diagnostic group was estimated by the average annual percent change (AAPC), as described in Chapter 2. Table 4.2 gives AAPCs for total cancers and ICCC-3 groups, and for subgroups that had an average of at least five cases per year during 1966–2000. In some of the subgroups, the first few years of registration were excluded from the analysis because the specificity of diagnosis had improved over time – there were decreases in large 'unspecified' categories which were balanced by increases in one or more specified categories, mainly during the first one or two five-year periods from 1966 (see Figs. 4.1–4.3). For each of these subgroups, the start of the analysis time was defined as the year following the last five-year period during which at least 6% of cases fell within the 'unspecified' category for the group: 1971 for leukaemia and lymphoma

Text starts on page 116

Table 4.1 Recorded incidence of childhood cancer by five-year period of diagnosis, Great Britain 1966–2000

Diagnostic groups and subgroups	Total number of cases	Age-standardized rate per million child-years (world standard)						
		1966–70	1971–75	1976–80	1981–85	1986–90	1991–95	1996–2000
ICCC-3 groups (in bold) and subgroups, excluding non-ICCC-2 diagnoses (see text)								
Leukaemias	**15476**	**35.57**	**39.65**	**40.49**	**39.51**	**42.40**	**43.18**	**45.53**
Lymphoid leukaemias	12033	23.42	30.49	32.95	31.98	34.05	35.45	36.80
Acute myeloid leukaemias	2465	5.44	6.92	6.07	6.00	6.45	6.41	6.79
Chronic myeloid leukaemias	228	0.51	0.57	0.59	0.43	0.65	0.41	0.68
Juvenile/chronic myelomonocytic leukaemias	128	0.07	0.40	0.21	0.45	0.41	0.39	0.77
Unspecified and other specified leukaemias	622	6.14	1.27	0.67	0.65	0.84	0.52	0.49
Lymphomas and reticuloendothelial neoplasms	**4796**	**10.46**	**10.18**	**11.57**	**10.92**	**11.58**	**12.19**	**12.85**
Hodgkin lymphomas	1959	3.70	3.96	4.56	4.67	4.46	4.65	5.29
Non-Hodgkin lymphomas (except Burkitt lymphoma)	2345	5.35	5.66	5.98	5.42	6.24	5.87	5.33
Burkitt lymphoma	281	0.10	0.15	0.36	0.42	0.58	1.34	2.11
Miscellaneous lymphoreticular neoplasms	69	0.10	0.19	0.49	0.22	0.10	0.11	0.04
Unspecified lymphomas	142	1.23	0.22	0.19	0.19	0.19	0.22	0.08
CNS and miscellaneous intracranial and intraspinal neoplasms	**11252**	**24.26**	**25.22**	**27.27**	**26.71**	**29.04**	**33.35**	**33.56**
Ependymomas and choroid plexus tumour	1223	2.90	3.16	3.53	3.22	2.92	3.31	3.61
Astrocytomas	4320	7.49	8.67	10.27	9.60	11.77	14.27	14.37
Intracranial and intraspinal embryonal tumours	2274	4.97	5.06	5.52	6.23	6.06	6.53	6.68
Other gliomas	1392	1.12	4.02	4.20	3.98	4.14	3.48	3.48

Other specified intracranial and intraspinal neoplasms	1105	1.81	1.96	2.66	2.14	2.42	3.85	4.12
Unspecified intracranial and intraspinal neoplasms	938	5.96	2.36	1.09	1.54	1.73	1.92	1.30
Neuroblastoma and other peripheral nervous cell tumours	**3083**	**8.68**	**7.93**	**7.42**	**8.32**	**10.08**	**8.84**	**9.85**
Neuroblastoma and ganglioneuroblastoma	3035	8.61	7.76	7.32	8.19	9.92	8.77	9.72
Other peripheral nervous cell tumours	48	0.08	0.17	0.10	0.13	0.16	0.07	0.13
Retinoblastoma	**1397**	**3.89**	**3.78**	**3.92**	**3.74**	**4.18**	**4.94**	**4.19**
Retinoblastoma	1397	3.89	3.78	3.92	3.74	4.18	4.94	4.19
Renal tumours	**2772**	**7.25**	**7.42**	**7.94**	**7.42**	**8.00**	**7.98**	**8.57**
Nephroblastoma and other nonepithelial renal tumours	2710	7.10	7.27	7.81	7.33	7.93	7.73	8.40
Renal carcinomas	53	0.14	0.11	0.10	0.09	0.07	0.20	0.12
Unspecified malignant renal tumours	9	0.02	0.04	0.02	0.00	0.00	0.04	0.05
Hepatic tumours	**393**	**0.78**	**0.82**	**1.03**	**1.06**	**1.25**	**1.30**	**1.52**
Hepatoblastoma	308	0.66	0.70	0.89	0.83	0.89	1.11	1.26
Hepatic carcinomas	83	0.12	0.12	0.14	0.23	0.34	0.19	0.24
Unspecified malignant hepatic tumours	2	0.00	0.00	0.00	0.00	0.02	0.00	0.02
Malignant bone tumours	**2105**	**3.90**	**4.43**	**5.06**	**5.10**	**5.18**	**4.91**	**4.65**
Osteosarcomas	1147	2.45	2.65	2.41	2.52	2.56	2.65	2.51
Chondrosarcomas	42	0.08	0.05	0.13	0.09	0.11	0.09	0.11
Ewing tumour and related bone sarcomas	793	1.02	1.40	2.22	2.25	2.21	1.88	1.85
Other specified malignant bone tumours	72	0.19	0.16	0.15	0.16	0.23	0.17	0.10

Table 4.1 (continued) Recorded incidence of childhood cancer by five-year period of diagnosis, Great Britain 1966–2000

Diagnostic groups and subgroups	Total number of cases	Age-standardized rate per million child-years (world standard)						
		1966–70	1971–75	1976–80	1981–85	1986–90	1991–95	1996–2000
ICCC-3 groups (in bold) and subgroups, excluding non-ICCC-2 diagnoses (see text)								
Unspecified malignant bone tumours	51	0.17	0.17	0.16	0.09	0.07	0.11	0.09
Soft tissue and other extraosseous sarcomas	**3040**	**5.82**	**6.67**	**6.87**	**7.64**	**8.86**	**10.15**	**9.17**
Rhabdomyosarcomas	1756	2.71	4.22	4.61	5.20	5.47	5.58	5.03
Fibrosarcomas, peripheral nerve sheath tumours and other fibrous neoplasms	328	1.26	0.79	0.61	0.76	0.78	0.77	0.69
Kaposi sarcoma	8	0.00	0.00	0.04	0.01	0.00	0.05	0.03
Other specified soft tissue sarcomas	690	0.82	0.95	1.01	1.28	1.92	3.28	2.85
Unspecified soft tissue sarcomas	258	1.03	0.71	0.60	0.40	0.70	0.46	0.57
Germ cell tumours, trophoblastic tumours and neoplasms of gonads	**1455**	**2.74**	**2.68**	**3.36**	**4.17**	**4.44**	**4.24**	**4.85**
Intracranial and intraspinal germ cell tumours	392	0.35	0.52	0.82	1.19	1.04	1.44	1.48
Malignant extracranial and extragonadal germ cell tumours	318	0.81	0.65	0.70	0.80	1.20	1.00	1.25
Malignant gonadal germ cell tumours	683	1.39	1.39	1.74	2.02	1.92	1.71	2.04
Gonadal carcinomas	45	0.14	0.04	0.07	0.09	0.25	0.07	0.07
Other and unspecified malignant gonadal tumours	17	0.05	0.07	0.01	0.06	0.04	0.02	0.02

Other malignant epithelial neoplasms and malignant melanomas	1382	2.33	2.09	2.72	3.27	3.92	4.02	4.31
Adrenocortical carcinomas	85	0.23	0.25	0.29	0.25	0.10	0.19	0.29
Thyroid carcinomas	201	0.29	0.33	0.38	0.45	0.53	0.45	0.75
Nasopharyngeal carcinomas	110	0.17	0.22	0.36	0.31	0.23	0.20	0.19
Malignant melanomas	358	0.45	0.31	0.72	0.79	1.11	1.53	1.18
Skin carcinomas	228	0.23	0.35	0.37	0.54	0.81	0.65	0.75
Other and unspecified carcinomas	400	0.96	0.64	0.61	0.94	1.14	1.00	1.14
Other and unspecified malignant neoplasms	**243**	**0.85**	**0.31**	**0.27**	**0.45**	**0.58**	**1.19**	**0.69**
Other specified malignant tumours	31	0.02	0.06	0.07	0.08	0.04	0.11	0.22
Other unspecified malignant tumours	212	0.84	0.25	0.20	0.37	0.54	1.08	0.47
Total cancers	**47,394**	**106.54**	**111.19**	**117.92**	**118.32**	**129.50**	**136.28**	**139.73**

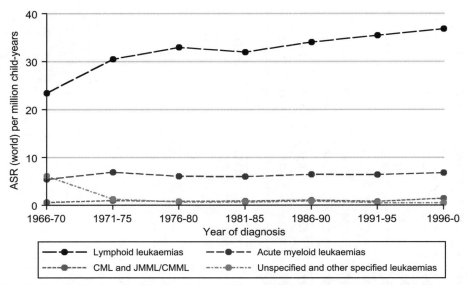

Fig. 4.1 Recorded incidence of leukaemias in children aged 0–14 years, by diagnostic subgroup and five-year calendar period of diagnosis. Great Britain, 1966–2000.

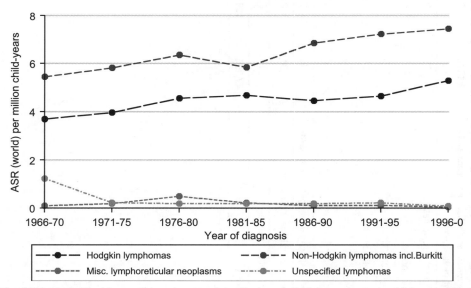

Fig. 4.2 Recorded incidence of lymphomas and reticuloendothelial neoplasms in children aged 0–14 years, by diagnostic subgroup and five-year calendar period of diagnosis. Great Britain, 1966–2000.

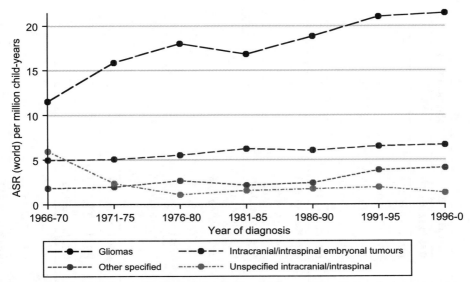

Fig. 4.3 Recorded incidence of CNS and miscellaneous intracranial and intraspinal neoplasms in children aged 0–14 years, by diagnostic group and five-year calendar period of diagnosis. Great Britain, 1966–2000.

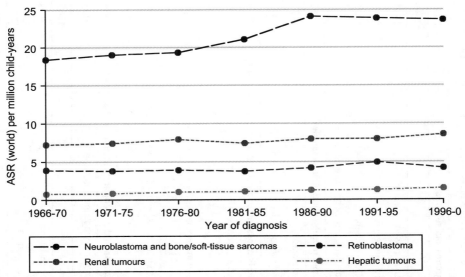

Fig. 4.4 Recorded incidence of neuroblastoma and other peripheral nervous cell tumours, malignant bone tumours, and soft tissue and other extraosseous sarcomas, combined; retinoblastoma; renal tumours; and hepatic tumours; in children aged 0–14 years, by diagnostic group and five-year calendar period of diagnosis. Great Britain, 1966–2000.

Table 4.2 Time trends in recorded incidence of childhood cancer from 1966, 1971, 1976 or 1986–2000, Great Britain

Diagnostic groups and subgroups	Start	Cases per year	AAPC (95% CI)	Significance tests
Leukaemias	**1966**	**442**	**0.68 (0.52 to 0.83)**	A *
Lymphoid leukaemias	1971	352	0.71 (0.49 to 0.93)	*
Acute myeloid leukaemias	1971	70	−0.06 (−0.54 to 0.42)	A
Chronic myeloid leukaemias	1971	6	0.71 (−0.87 to 2.33)	A
Unspecified and other specified leukaemias	1971	7	−3.46 (−4.90 to −2.01)	#
Lymphomas and reticuloendothelial neoplasms	**1966**	**137**	**0.74 (0.46 to 1.02)**	A *
Hodgkin lymphomas	1971	57	0.89 (0.35 to 1.43)	S *
Non-Hodgkin lymphomas including Burkitt lymphoma	1971	75	1.06 (0.59 to 1.53)	A *
CNS and miscellaneous intracranial and intraspinal neoplasms	**1966**	**321**	**1.16 (0.98 to 1.34)**	S *
Ependymomas and choroid plexus tumour	1976	33	0.18 (−0.74 to 1.12)	
Astrocytomas	1976	131	2.17 (1.69 to 2.65)	*
Intracranial and intraspinal embryonal tumours	1976	65	0.81 (0.15 to 1.48)	*
Other gliomas	1976	42	−1.00 (−1.81 to −0.18)	*
Other specified intracranial and intraspinal neoplasms	1976	34	3.13 (2.19 to 4.09)	#
Unspecified intracranial and intraspinal neoplasms	1976	16	1.21 (−0.13 to 2.57)	#
Neuroblastoma and other peripheral nervous cell tumours	**1966**	**88**	**0.50 (0.15 to 0.84)**	# A *
Neuroblastoma and ganglioneuroblastoma	1966	86	0.50 (0.15 to 0.84)	# A
Retinoblastoma	**1966**	**39**	**0.60 (0.10 to 1.12)**	*
Unilateral retinoblastoma	1966	24	0.78 (0.13 to 1.43)	A *
Bilateral retinoblastoma	1966	14	0.19 (−0.65 to 1.05)	A
Renal tumours	**1966**	**79**	**0.45 (0.09 to 0.81)**	*
Nephroblastoma and other nonepithelial renal tumours	1966	77	0.44 (0.08 to 0.81)	*

	Start year	Cases	AAPC (95% CI)	A	#	*
Hepatic tumours	1966	11	**2.16 (1.17 to 3.15)**			*
Hepatoblastoma	1966	8	1.99 (0.89 to 3.11)			*
Malignant bone tumours	1966	60	**0.52 (0.09 to 0.94)**			*
Osteosarcomas	1966	32	0.08 (−0.50 to 0.66)	A		*
Ewing tumour and related bone sarcomas	1966	22	1.44 (0.75 to 2.14)			*
Soft tissue and other extraosseous sarcomas	1966	86	**1.81 (1.45 to 2.16)**	A		*
Germ cell tumours, trophoblastic tumours and neoplasms of gonads	1966	41	**2.06 (1.54 to 2.57)**	A	#	*
Intracranial and intraspinal germ cell tumours	1976	13	2.90 (1.40 to 4.42)		#	*
Malignant extracranial and extragonadal germ cell tumours	1966	9	1.78 (0.69 to 2.87)			*
Malignant gonadal germ cell tumours: males	1966	9	0.99 (−0.05 to 2.04)		#	
Malignant gonadal germ cell tumours: females	1966	9	1.37 (0.32 to 2.44)			*
Other malignant epithelial neoplasms and malignant melanomas	1966	39	**2.53 (2.00 to 3.07)**			*
Thyroid carcinomas	1986	6	3.42 (−1.17 to 8.22)			
Malignant melanomas	1966	10	4.49 (3.39 to 5.61)			*
Other and unspecified carcinomas	1986	12	0.42 (−2.81 to 3.74)			
Other and unspecified malignant neoplasms	1966	6	**1.75 (0.50 to 3.01)**		#	*
Total cancers	1966	1354	**0.95 (0.86 to 1.04)**			*

ICCC-3 diagnostic groups (in bold) and subgroups with at least five cases per year, excluding non-ICCC-2 diagnoses (see text)

Analysis period is from start year to 2000

Average number of cases per year during analysis period (rounded down to the nearest whole number)

Average annual% change (AAPC) with 95% confidence interval (95% CI), based on Poisson model allowing for age group and sex (see text)

Test for lack of fit to the Poisson model: p < 0.05. Estimated confidence interval and other test results may be inaccurate (see text)

A Test for difference in trend between age groups: p < 0.05

S Test for difference in trend between boys and girls: p < 0.05

* Test for trend: p < 0.05

subgroups, 1976 for intracranial and intraspinal neoplasms (including intracranial and intraspinal germ cell tumours), and 1986 for carcinomas. Soft-tissue sarcoma subgroups were not analysed, because there may have been diagnostic shift between them in the past, and there was a fairly high proportion of unspecified tumours even in recent years. Skin carcinomas were not analysed because there are known ascertainment problems for this subgroup. The emergence of specified Burkitt lymphoma over time is certainly due to classification change, and so it was combined with the main non-Hodgkin lymphoma subgroup. Trends in gonadal germ cell tumours were analysed separately for boys and girls because the age distributions are completely different (see Fig. 3.33), and it seemed reasonable to expect that the trend might vary by both age group and sex. Confidence intervals for the AAPCs and the results of tests for differences in trend by age group or sex are given in Table 4.2. For some diagnostic groups, as shown, these may be inaccurate because there was evidence that the necessary assumptions might not be valid (see Chapter 2), but the AAPC itself should be reliable as an estimate of average change.

Table 4.3 presents separate five-yearly incidence rates and AAPCs by age group, or by sex, where there was a statistically significant difference (at the 5% level) in trend between age groups, or between boys and girls, for any of the diagnostic groups or subgroups shown in Table 4.2. Table 4.4 gives the same information for all cancers combined.

4.2 Results

4.2.1 Leukaemias

Between 1966 and 2000, the recorded incidence of childhood leukaemia increased by 0.68% per year on average (95% confidence interval (CI) 0.52 to 0.83). This was driven by an increase in the largest subgroup, lymphoid leukaemia (ALL), for which the AAPC was 0.71% (CI 0.49 to 0.93) from 1971 to 2000. Overall there was no significant change in the other main subgroup, acute myeloid leukaemia (AML): the AAPC 1971–2000 was –0.06% (CI –0.54 to 0.42). There was no statistically significant overall trend in CML. During 1971–2000 there was a decrease (AAPC –3.46%) in 'unspecified and other specified leukaemias', showing that some improvement in specificity was still continuing after 1970, but the number of cases involved was relatively small (see Fig. 4.1). There were no statistically significant differences between boys and girls in the leukaemia trends. In AML and CML, there were statistically significant differences between age groups. AML rates increased significantly at age 0 (AAPC 1.85%, CI 0.36 to 3.35), but not in the other age groups. There was a very large decrease in CML diagnosed at age 0 (AAPC –17.27%, CI –30.63 to –1.34), but this was based on only 5 cases.

4.2.2 Lymphomas and reticuloendothelial neoplasms

Recorded incidence of lymphomas increased by 0.74% per year on average from 1966 to 2000 (CI 0.46 to 1.02). From 1971 to 2000, there were statistically significant increases in both Hodgkin lymphomas (AAPC 0.89%, CI 0.35 to 1.43) and non-Hodgkin lymphomas including Burkitt lymphomas (NHL) (AAPC 1.06, CI 0.59 to 1.53). There were significant differences in trend between age groups. For lymphomas as a whole, there was

Text starts on page 121

Table 4.3 Time trends in recorded incidence of childhood cancer, by age group or sex, for diagnoses in which the trend differed significantly by age group or sex (see Table 4.2), from 1966 or 1971–2000, Great Britain

Cases per year	Group	Rate per million child-years, by five-year period of diagnosis							AAPC (95% CI)	Significance tests
		1966–70	1971–75	1976–80	1981–85	1986–90	1991–95	1996–2000		
Acute myeloid leukaemias										
8	Age 0	–	9.13	9.72	10.07	11.38	12.98	13.98	1.85 (0.36 to 3.35)	*
22	Age 1–4	–	7.99	7.20	7.50	8.18	7.22	8.67	0.22 (–0.63 to 1.07)	
17	Age 5–9	–	5.87	4.38	4.27	4.24	4.09	4.66	–0.81 (–1.76 to 0.15)	
22	Age 10–14	–	6.36	5.78	5.24	5.73	6.38	5.23	–0.40 (–1.26 to 0.47)	
Chronic myeloid leukaemias										
< 1	Age 0	–	0.52	0.91	0.00	0.00	0.00	0.00	–17.27 (–30.63 to –1.34)	*
1	Age 1–4	–	0.42	0.52	0.37	0.70	0.27	0.28	–0.89 (–4.44 to 2.80)	
1	Age 5–9	–	0.49	0.39	0.36	0.76	0.33	0.64	1.26 (–1.66 to 4.28)	#
3	Age 10–14	–	0.84	0.80	0.69	0.66	0.75	1.32	1.72 (–0.56 to 4.05)	#
Lymphomas and reticuloendothelial neoplasms										
1	Age 0	3.34	3.65	5.17	1.44	1.08	1.08	1.16	–4.43 (–6.86 to –1.93)	*
22	Age 1–4	7.49	7.10	7.35	7.28	7.48	7.62	8.17	0.29 (–0.38 to 0.97)	
45	Age 5–9	10.51	10.58	12.64	10.28	12.21	12.71	13.07	0.70 (0.22 to 1.19)	*
67	Age 10–14	15.48	14.77	16.59	18.03	18.04	19.44	20.71	1.08 (0.67 to 1.49)	*
Hodgkin lymphomas										
39	Males	–	5.29	6.52	6.33	5.80	6.30	6.58	0.51 (–0.14 to 1.17)	
18	Females	–	2.57	2.48	2.93	3.05	2.92	3.93	1.69 (0.73 to 2.66)	*

Table 4.3 (continued) Time trends in recorded incidence of childhood cancer, by age group or sex, for diagnoses in which the trend differed significantly by age group or sex (see Table 4.2), from 1966 or 1971–2000, Great Britain

Group	Cases per year	Rate per million child-years, by five-year period of diagnosis							AAPC (95% CI)	Significance tests
		1966–70	1971–75	1976–80	1981–85	1986–90	1991–95	1996–2000		
Non-Hodgkin lymphomas including Burkitt lymphoma										
Age 0	1	–	3.13	2.74	0.86	0.54	0.81	0.87	−6.61 (−10.60 to −2.44)	*
Age 1–4	16	–	5.31	5.20	5.51	5.94	6.15	6.55	0.95 (−0.05 to 1.95)	
Age 5–9	28	–	6.31	7.97	6.01	8.02	7.74	9.27	1.14 (0.38 to 1.90)	*
Age 10–14	29	–	6.50	6.72	7.31	8.12	9.46	8.10	1.31 (0.55 to 2.08)	*
CNS and miscellaneous intracranial and intraspinal neoplasms										
Males	174	26.31	27.51	28.80	28.63	30.56	33.96	35.31	0.98 (0.74 to 1.23)	*
Females	146	22.11	22.81	25.66	24.69	27.44	32.71	31.73	1.37 (1.10 to 1.64)	*
Neuroblastoma and other peripheral nervous cell tumours										
Age 0	23	27.85	26.60	27.05	35.38	35.22	33.27	39.02	1.16 (0.50 to 1.84)	*
Age 1–4	47	14.33	13.24	13.44	14.92	19.09	16.71	18.25	1.07 (0.61 to 1.54)	*
Age 5–9	12	4.54	3.69	2.61	2.41	3.84	2.71	3.27	−1.05 (−1.94 to −0.14)	*
Age 10–14	4	2.15	2.00	1.11	0.64	0.72	0.75	0.44	−5.54 (−7.21 to −3.84)	*
Neuroblastoma and ganglioneuroblastoma										
Age 0	23	27.85	26.34	27.05	35.09	34.95	33.27	39.02	1.17 (0.50 to 1.85)	*
Age 1–4	46	14.33	12.94	13.30	14.92	18.74	16.64	18.04	1.06 (0.59 to 1.54)	*
Age 5–9	12	4.49	3.56	2.56	2.35	3.84	2.60	3.16	−1.11 (−2.02 to −0.20)	*
Age 10–14	3	1.94	1.95	0.98	0.35	0.60	0.70	0.33	−6.18 (−7.99 to −4.33)	# *
Unilateral retinoblastoma										
Age 0	5	5.79	6.00	8.21	6.33	8.40	11.09	10.77	2.30 (0.94 to 3.68)	*

	N								AAPC (95% CI)	#	*
Age 1–4	17	5.81	6.26	4.98	4.41	6.22	6.28	5.64	0.14 (−0.63 to 0.91)		
Age 5–14	1	0.20	0.09	0.26	0.14	0.35	0.31	0.24	2.25 (−0.28 to 4.84)	#	*
Bilateral retinoblastoma											
Age 0	9	12.03	8.61	14.59	15.53	12.73	15.15	13.69	0.81 (−0.23 to 1.85)		
Age 1–14	4	0.59	0.54	0.27	0.40	0.35	0.68	0.27	−1.07 (−2.54 to 0.43)	#	
Osteosarcomas											
Age 0–4	<1	0.22	0.24	0.12	0.18	0.11	0.21	0.06	−1.92 (−5.87 to 2.19)		
Age 5–9	7	1.62	1.78	1.72	1.32	2.15	2.49	2.30	1.35 (0.15 to 2.56)	#	*
Age 10–14	24	6.35	6.83	6.23	6.97	6.27	6.09	6.00	−0.27 (−0.93 to 0.40)		
Soft tissue and other extraosseous sarcomas											
Age 0	9	10.70	12.78	11.85	12.66	13.27	14.88	14.56	0.91 (−0.14 to 1.96)	#	
Age 1–4	28	7.60	8.59	7.72	9.26	11.47	11.83	10.29	1.44 (0.84 to 2.05)		*
Age 5–9	24	4.72	4.80	6.10	6.25	6.34	8.29	7.87	1.86 (1.19 to 2.53)		*
Age 10–14	24	3.83	5.06	5.47	6.13	7.70	9.17	7.99	2.59 (1.90 to 3.28)		*
Germ cell tumours, trophoblastic tumours and neoplasms of gonads											
Age 0	6	8.47	6.00	6.69	9.49	11.38	9.20	13.40	1.80 (0.55 to 3.07)		*
Age 1–4	12	3.37	3.40	4.61	4.70	5.45	4.21	4.23	0.93 (0.03 to 1.83)	#	*
Age 5–9	6	0.74	1.47	1.38	1.98	1.51	2.16	2.25	2.56 (1.23 to 3.90)		*
Age 10–14	15	2.78	2.37	3.34	4.60	4.78	5.28	6.11	2.96 (2.10 to 3.83)	#	*

Average number of cases per year during analysis period (rounded down to the nearest whole number)

Rate per million child-years, for grouped year of diagnosis during analysis period

Separate rates for males and females are age-standardized to the world standard population

Average annual% change (AAPC) with 95% confidence interval (95% CI), based on Poisson model allowing for age group and sex (see text)

Test for lack of fit to the Poisson model: $p < 0.05$. Estimated confidence interval may be inaccurate (see text)

* Test for trend: $p < 0.05$

Table 4.4 Time trends in total recorded incidence of childhood cancer, by age group and by sex, Great Britain 1966–2000

Group	Total number of cases	1966–70	1971–75	1976–80	1981–85	1986–90	1991–95	1996–2000	AAPC (95% CI)
		Age-specific rate per million child-years, by diagnosis period							
Age 0	4085	138.60	133.54	144.05	157.91	164.99	177.44	193.07	1.18 (0.88 to 1.48)
Age 1–4	17,577	145.63	155.02	162.14	161.05	178.28	180.33	188.32	0.84 (0.70 to 0.98)
Age 5–9	12,841	81.68	88.67	94.85	90.51	99.07	106.18	108.40	0.90 (0.73 to 1.07)
Age 10–14	12,891	83.93	83.49	89.41	93.09	101.83	111.77	108.50	1.08 (0.90 to 1.25)
		Age-standardized rate per million child-years (world standard population), by diagnosis period							
Males	26,384	114.79	123.60	128.77	127.79	138.76	147.59	151.10	0.91 (0.79 to 1.03)
Females	21,010	97.89	98.10	106.46	108.35	119.78	124.46	127.80	1.00 (0.86 to 1.13)
Children	47,394	106.54	111.19	117.92	118.32	129.50	136.28	139.73	0.95 (0.86 to 1.04)

Excludes non-ICCC-2 diagnoses (see text). All trends are statistically significant ($p < 0.05$) and there is no evidence of lack of fit a decreasing trend at age 0 of −4.43% (CI −6.86 to −1.93) from 1966 to 2000, based on a relatively small number of cases; there was no significant trend in age group 1–4, but increases in age groups 5–9 (AAPC 0.70%, CI 0.22 to 1.19) and 10–14 (AAPC 1.08%, CI 0.67 to 1.49). A similar pattern appeared in NHL during 1971–2000: there was a decrease at age 0 (AAPC −6.61%, CI −10.60 to −2.44), and increases in age groups 5–9 (AAPC 1.14%, CI 0.38 to 1.90) and 10–14 (AAPC 1.31%, CI 0.55 to 2.08). For Hodgkin lymphomas, there was a statistically significant difference in trend between boys and girls. The increase in rates for boys was not statistically significant (AAPC 0.51%, CI −0.14 to 1.17); the increase for girls was larger and significant (AAPC 1.69%, CI 0.73 to 2.66).

4.2.3 CNS and miscellaneous intracranial and intraspinal neoplasms

As a whole, this disparate group increased by 1.16% per year on average from 1966 to 2000 (CI 0.98 to 1.34). From 1976 to 2000, there were statistically significant increases in two subgroups: astrocytomas (AAPC 2.17%, CI 1.69 to 2.65) and intracranial and intraspinal embryonal tumours (AAPC 0.81%, CI 0.15 to 1.48); there was also a large increase in 'other specified intracranial and intraspinal neoplasms' (AAPC 3.13%). There was no significant trend in 'ependymomas and choroid plexus tumour' (AAPC 0.18%, CI −0.74 to 1.12). There was a significant decrease in 'other gliomas' (AAPC −1.00%, CI −1.81 to −0.18). Since this category includes unspecified gliomas, the decrease probably represents improvements in specificity within the broad diagnosis of glioma, and is likely to explain part of the increase in astrocytoma. The looser category 'unspecified intracranial and intraspinal neoplasms', however, did not decrease during 1976–2000 (AAPC 1.21%). There was a statistically significant difference in trend between boys and girls for the group of CNS tumours as a whole from 1966 to 2000: the increase was larger for girls (AAPC 1.37%, CI 1.10 to 1.64) than for boys (AAPC 0.98%, CI 0.74 to 1.23). There were no significant differences in trend between age groups.

4.2.4 Neuroblastoma and other peripheral nervous cell tumours

There was a small increasing trend in 'neuroblastoma and ganglioneuroblastoma' 1966–2000 (AAPC 0.50%). There was no difference in trend between boys and girls, but there were large differences between age groups. The overall increase derived entirely from the younger children: age 0 (AAPC 1.17%, CI 0.50 to 1.85) and age 1–4 (AAPC 1.06%, CI 0.59 to 1.54). There was a decrease in age group 5–9 (AAPC −1.11%, CI −2.02 to −0.20) and a sharp decrease in age group 10–14 (AAPC −6.18%), based on a small number of cases.

4.2.5 Retinoblastoma

Overall, there was an increasing trend in retinoblastoma 1966–2000 (AAPC 0.60%, CI 0.10 to 1.12). This was apparently due to an increase in unilateral retinoblastoma (AAPC 0.78%, CI 0.13 to 1.43); there was no statistically significant trend in bilateral retinoblastoma (AAPC 0.19%, CI −0.65 to 1.05). However, both types had significantly different trends in different age groups. There was a large increase in unilateral retinoblastoma at age 0 (AAPC 2.30%, CI 0.94 to 3.68) but no significant increase in age group 1–4 (AAPC 0.14%, CI –0.63 to 0.91). In bilateral retinoblastoma there was a tendency for rates at age 0 to increase (AAPC 0.81%, CI –0.23 to 1.85), and rates in children aged 1–14 to decrease (AAPC –1.07%). There were no differences in trend between boys and girls.

4.2.6 Renal tumours

There was a small just-significant increasing trend in 'nephroblastoma and other nonepithelial renal tumours' 1966–2000 (AAPC 0.44%, CI 0.08 to 0.81). There were no statistically significant differences by age group or sex.

4.2.7 Hepatic tumours

There was an increasing trend in hepatic tumours 1966–2000 (AAPC 2.16%, CI 1.17 to 3.15), ascribed mainly to hepatoblastoma (AAPC 1.99%, CI 0.89 to 3.11). There were no statistically significant differences by age group or sex.

4.2.8 Malignant bone tumours

Overall, there was a just-significant increasing trend 1966–2000 in this group (AAPC 0.52%, CI 0.09 to 0.94). This was due to an increase in 'Ewing tumour and related bone sarcomas' (AAPC 1.44%, CI 0.75 to 2.14). There was no apparent change in osteosarcoma (AAPC 0.08%, CI –0.50 to 0.66). There were no statistically significant differences in trend between boys and girls, but for osteosarcoma there were significant differences between age groups. The rates increased in children aged 5–9 (AAPC 1.35%), but not in older children (AAPC –0.27%, CI –0.93 to 0.40).

4.2.9 Soft tissue and other extraosseous sarcomas

There was a statistically significant increasing trend 1966–2000 overall (AAPC 1.81%, CI 1.45 to 2.16). Subgroups were not analysed. There were no statistically significant differences in trend between boys and girls, but there were differences between age groups, with a tendency for larger increases in older children. The largest increase was in age group 10–14 (AAPC 2.59%, CI 1.90 to 3.28), and the smallest was at age 0 (AAPC 0.91%).

4.2.10 Germ cell tumours, trophoblastic tumours and neoplasms of gonads

For consistency, this group was analysed in the same way as the other main ICCC-3 groups. During 1966–2000 there was an overall increasing trend (AAPC 2.06%), and different trends between age groups, with a tendency for larger increases in older children. However, the group combines diagnoses that perhaps should not be analysed together, and the periods for subgroup analysis vary because there is no single 'unspecified' category. During 1976–2000, there was a large increase in 'intracranial and intraspinal germ cell tumours' (AAPC 2.90%). Analysis for this subgroup, like the subgroups of the main 'CNS and intracranial and intraspinal' group, was restricted to the more recent time period because of the high proportion of 'unspecified intracranial and intraspinal neoplasms' in the earlier years. There were no significant differences by age group or sex.

Gonadal germ cell tumours were analysed separately for boys and girls. During 1976–2000, the increasing trend was apparently larger for girls (AAPC 1.37%, CI 0.32 to 2.44) than for boys (AAPC 0.99%). There were no significant differences in trend by age group.

4.2.11 Other malignant epithelial neoplasms and malignant melanomas

During 1966–2000, there was a statistically significant increase in this group overall (AAPC 2.53%, CI 2.00 to 3.07). This was partly due to a large increase in malignant melanomas 1966–2000 (AAPC 4.49%, CI 3.39 to 5.61). There also appeared to be a tendency for thyroid carcinomas to increase, but this was not statistically significant over the relatively short analysis period 1986–2000 (AAPC 3.42%, CI −1.17 to 8.22). There was no significant change in the miscellaneous subgroup 'other and unspecified carcinomas' during 1986–2000 (AAPC 0.42%, CI −2.81 to 3.74). There were no significant differences in trend between age groups or between boys and girls.

4.2.12 Other and unspecified malignant neoplasms

There was an increasing trend during 1966–2000 (AAPC 1.75%), which did not differ by age group or sex.

4.2.13 Total cancers

Between 1966 and 2000, the total recorded incidence of childhood cancer increased by 0.95% per year on average (CI 0.86 to 1.04). There was a larger increase in age groups 0 and 10–14 than in the other age groups, and a slightly larger increase in girls than in boys, but these differences were not statistically significant.

4.3 Discussion

In this analysis, the recorded incidence of childhood cancer increased by 0.9% per year on average over the 35-year study period, equivalent to a total increase of 38% from 1966 to 2000. There was an increase in each of the twelve main diagnostic groups of ICCC-3, varying between groups from 0.5 to 2.5% per year. There were also statistically significant increases in most of the subgroups of ICCC-3.

There were some exceptions to this pattern. In particular there was no significant overall change in the subgroups AML, 'ependymoma and choroid plexus tumour' and osteosarcoma over the periods analysed (1971–2000, 1976–2000 and 1966–2000, respectively), and there were decreases in 'unspecified and other specified leukaemias' (1971–2000) and in 'other gliomas' (1976–2000), a category which consists mainly of unspecified gliomas. The decreases in the 'unspecified' categories reflect improvements in the specificity of diagnosis within ICCC-3 groups, but can explain only small proportions of the increases in other subgroups over the limited time periods analysed.

Within several diagnostic groups and subgroups there were statistically significant differences in trend between age groups, notably AML, NHL, neuroblastoma, retinoblastoma and osteosarcoma. In CNS tumours and Hodgkin lymphoma, there was a significant sex difference: for both, the increase was greater for girls than boys.

The results presented here are consistent with estimates from the Manchester Children's Tumour Registry (MCTR), a high-quality specialist population-based registry covering a region of North West England (McNally *et al.*, 2001a,b). Figures 4.5–4.8 compare MCTR and NRCT age-standardized incidence rates for broad diagnostic groups during the common time period. For the period 1954–98, the MCTR found statistically significant increases in ALL (AAPC 0.7% (0.2–1.1)), Hodgkin lymphoma (AAPC 1.2% (0.1–2.4)), CNS tumours (AAPC 0.9% (0.5–1.4), girls more than boys), and non-CNS solid tumours (AAPC 0.8% (0.4–1.2)), particularly germ cell tumours (AAPC 2.6% (1.2–4.0)). There was no statistically significant change in AML. All these are similar to the corresponding NRCT results. Unlike the NRCT, the MCTR found only a small increase in NHL, which was not statistically significant. The difference might be explained by aetiology, or it may simply be due to chance – for this group and for comparable groups in general, the NRCT AAPC estimate was well within the MCTR 95% CI.

In the present analysis, the trend estimates for total leukaemia by separate age groups (not shown in Table 4.3 because they were not significantly different from each other) were: AAPC 1.0% (0.3–1.6) at age 0, 0.8% (0.6–1.0) in age group 1–4, 0.6% (0.3–0.9) in age group 5–9 and 0.3% (–0.0 to 0.6) in age group 10–14. An age- and sex-specific analysis of leukaemia time trends in the NRCT data for Britain over the earlier period 1953–91 (Draper *et al.*, 1994) produced rather different results: for total leukaemia the AAPC was 0.5% for both boys and girls at age 0, 1.0% for boys and 0.9% for girls in age group 1–4, –0.1% for boys and 0.2% for girls in age group 5–9, and 0.0% (restricted to 1956–91) for boys and girls in age group 10–14. However, that analysis is not directly comparable with the present one, because mortality data were used to represent leukaemia incidence before 1962. Except for age group 5–9, the estimates fall within the 95% CI from the present analysis, as do almost all the age-specific results given in the same publication for comparable groups of solid tumours over the period 1962–91. The trend estimate obtained from an analysis (dos Santos Silva *et al.*, 1999) of NRCT data for testicular germ cell malignancies diagnosed under the age of 15 in England and Wales during 1962–95, AAPC 1.3% (0.2–2.5), was higher than the estimate for male gonadal germ cell tumours presented here, AAPC 0.99% (–0.05 to 2.04), but consistent, given the different time period and geographical area.

The largest published analyses of childhood cancer incidence trends are from consortia of high-quality population-based cancer registries: ACCIS (for regions within 15 European countries, including data for the whole of Britain) and SEER (for selected regions in the USA). The ACCIS studies found a 1.0% annual increase in all cancers combined during 1970–99 (Steliarova-Foucher *et al.*, 2004), and 1.1% during 1978–97 (Kaatsch *et al.*, 2006) – both similar to the results presented here, although the time periods are different. For 1978–97, the ACCIS study also analysed trends by European region. There was an increase of 1.1% in the data for the British Isles (which contributed 30.5% of all the cases) and there were similar increases in data from registries within (not necessarily the whole of) countries in other parts of Europe: East (represented by Estonia,

Text starts on page 127

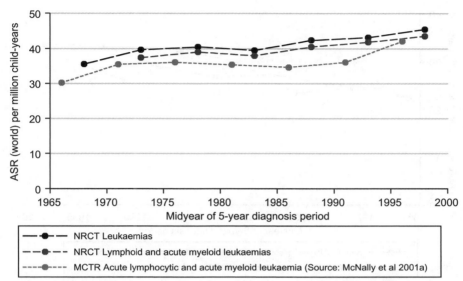

Fig. 4.5 Recorded incidence of leukaemias in children aged 0–14 years, by five-year calendar period of diagnosis. Comparison between Manchester Children's Tumour Registry (MCTR) 1964–98, and National Registry of Childhood Tumours (NRCT) 1966–2000.

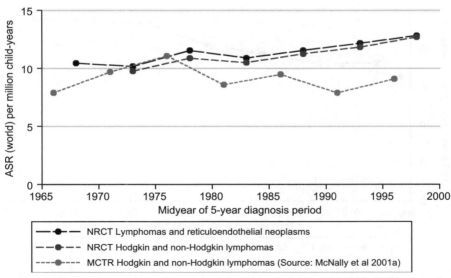

Fig. 4.6 Recorded incidence of lymphomas (and reticuloenthelial neoplasms) in children aged 0–14 years, by five-year calendar period of diagnosis. Comparison between Manchester Children's Tumour Registry (MCTR) 1964–98, and National Registry of Childhood Tumours (NRCT) 1966–2000.

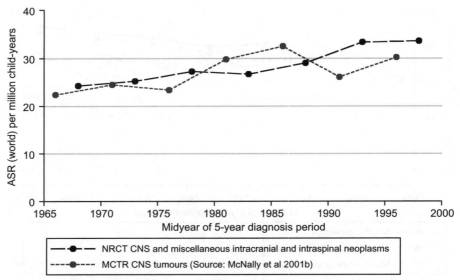

Fig. 4.7 Recorded incidence of CNS tumours (and miscellaneous intracranial and intraspinal neo-plasms) in children aged 0–14 years, by five-year calendar period of diagnosis. Comparison between Manchester Children's Tumour Registry (MCTR) 1964–98, and National Registry of Childhood Tumours (NRCT) 1966–2000.

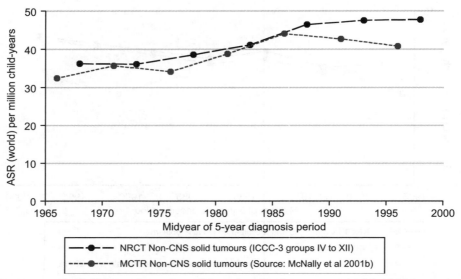

Fig. 4.8 Recorded incidence of non-CNS solid tumours (ICCC-3 groups IV–XII) in children aged 0–14 years, by five-year calendar period of diagnosis. Comparison between Manchester Children's Tumour Registry (MCTR) 1964–98, and National Registry of Childhood Tumours (NRCT) 1966–2000.

Hungary and Slovakia) 1.4%, North (Denmark, Finland, Iceland and Norway) 1.0%, South (Italy, Slovenia and Spain) 1.2%, West (France, Netherlands, Switzerland and Germany) 1.1%. The SEER analysis of trends in nine areas of the USA (San Francisco, Connecticut, Detroit, Hawaii, Iowa, New Mexico, Seattle, Utah and Atlanta) (Ries *et al.*, 2006) found a smaller increase, 0.6%, during 1975–2003.

Table 4.5 compares results from NRCT, ACCIS and SEER, over varying time periods, for the main diagnostic groups. All these studies found increases in all or most of the diagnostic groups. For the largest group, leukaemias, the rates of increase were similar, 0.6–0.7%. For two groups, there were increases of more than 1% per year in all three studies: CNS tumours (1.2–1.7%) and germ cell tumours (1.0–2.1%). Within each study, there was relatively little change in bone tumours and a relatively large increase in epithelial neoplasms and melanomas, compared to other diagnostic groups. There were some notable differences between studies, particularly in neuroblastoma (increasing more rapidly in the ACCIS study than in either SEER or the NRCT) and lymphomas (increasing in NRCT and ACCIS but not SEER). However, the different time periods and population sizes have to be remembered.

In all three studies, the range of different trends within diagnostic groups and subgroups appears to be superimposed on a background tendency for recorded incidence rates to increase. One obvious possible explanation is that notification of diagnosed cases to the NRCT and other registries may have become more complete over time. The general move towards more centralized treatment of childhood cancer has facilitated registration everywhere. In Britain, the UKCCSG (2002) now provides an additional mechanism for recording new patients. However, the national cancer registration system is backed by death registration, which is essentially complete, and the ascertainment rate of known patients to the NRCT is believed to be high. Completeness of registration of leukaemia and NHL in the NRCT during 1974–83 was estimated as 99% (Draper *et al.*, 1991), although, as the authors explained, the method used may over-estimate completeness because of the rather strong assumption that sources of ascertainment are independent. The NRCT recorded incidence rates presented here are generally not lower than the corresponding rates from the MCTR (Figs. 4.5–4.8), and ascertainment to the MCTR is thought to have been close to 100% for 45 years; a study of MCTR cases diagnosed in 1972–73 concluded that practically all children resident in the region who presented with life-threatening neoplasms were ascertained (Leck *et al.*, 1976). In general, for most diagnostic groups, if cancers were missed it seems more likely that they were never diagnosed than that they were diagnosed and not recorded.

In Britain and elsewhere, there were great improvements in the management of childhood cancer from the 1960s onwards (UKCCSG, 2002). The existence of effective new treatment protocols became an incentive to refer patients to specialist centres for diagnosis, and to develop better diagnostic techniques. If some childhood cancers were previously under-diagnosed, an increase in the reported incidence rate would be expected. For example, it has been convincingly argued that the introduction of magnetic resonance imaging (MRI) in the USA probably contributed to the increase in the reported incidence rate of childhood primary malignant brain tumours seen in the SEER registries in

Table 4.5 International comparison of time trends in recorded incidence of childhood cancer

Registry or group of registries	ACCIS	NRCT	SEER
Setting	Europe	Britain	USA
Time period	1978–97	1966–2000	1975–2003
Diagnostic group (ICCC-3)			
Leukaemias, myeloproliferative and myelodysplastic diseases	*0.6	*0.7	*0.6
Lymphomas and reticuloendothelial neoplasms	*0.9	*0.7	−0.4
CNS and miscellaneous intracranial and intraspinal neoplasms	*1.7	*1.2	*1.2
Neuroblastoma and other peripheral nervous cell tumours	*1.7	*0.5	0.2
Retinoblastoma	0.5	*0.6	0.6
Renal tumours	*0.8	*0.5	0.3
Hepatic tumours	0.8	*2.2	x
Malignant bone tumours	−0.3	*0.5	−0.1
Soft tissue and other extraosseous sarcomas	*1.8	*1.8	0.6
Germ cell tumours, trophoblastic tumours and neoplasms of gonads	*1.6	*2.1	1.0
Other malignant epithelial neoplasms and malignant melanomas	*1.3	*2.5	*0.8
Other and unspecified malignant neoplasms	1.1	*1.8	x
Total cancers	*1.1	*0.9	*0.6
Approximate average number of cases per year	**3900**	**1400**	**< 1000**

Average annual% change, over varying time periods as shown

x: statistic not reported

* Significance test for trend: $p < 0.05$

the mid-1980s (Black, 1998; Smith *et al.*, 1998). So the introduction and refinement of diagnostic imaging, particularly computerized tomography (CT) from the 1970s, and MRI from the 1980s, is probably a factor in the increase in reported CNS tumour rates seen in the NRCT and ACCIS. Previously some of these tumours, particularly the less aggressive ones, might have been diagnosed after the age of 15, or never. In the NRCT there was a larger increase in astrocytomas (AAPC 2.17%), a subgroup which includes a substantial proportion of low-grade tumours, than in embryonal CNS tumours (AAPC 0.81%), which are usually aggressive. A similar argument may apply to other cancers, particularly the less acute forms, and to other diagnostic techniques. For example, there is a rather striking plateau in the combined recorded incidence of neuroblastoma and tumours of bone and soft tissue from 1986–90 onwards (Fig. 4.4) – it is tempting to speculate that this might represent complete registration of these cancers following previous under-diagnosis. However, interpretation on these lines would need to take into account the possible effects of a change in the proportion of asymptomatic neuroblastomas diagnosed incidentally, and of shifts in the definition of malignancy for soft tissue neoplasms.

As diagnostic methods improve it becomes possible to classify disease more accurately. The gradual transfer of recorded incidence from less specific to more specific categories is an obvious effect – for example in gliomas and leukaemia before the mid-1970s. As described above, some of the subgroup analyses presented here cover limited time periods in an attempt to avoid this problem. Another possible effect is transfer between apparently specific categories – even perhaps neuroblastoma, lymphoma and tumours of bone and soft tissue (Cohn, 1999) – which in fact could not be clearly separated in the past. For example, before the development of special stains it was difficult to distinguish between types of soft tissue sarcoma, and fibrosarcoma was more often diagnosed than it would be now (Daugaard, 2004).

Any of the factors discussed above may explain some of the differences in trend between age groups that are shown in Table 4.3. For any diagnostic group, changes over time in completeness, accuracy or specificity of registration might vary with the age of the child, and so might produce artificially different time trends in different age groups. The anomalous trends in several leukaemia and lymphoma subgroups at age 0 probably represent uncertainty in diagnosis continuing for some time later in infants than in older children. For instance, although CML has been known to occur in infancy (Boque and Wilson, 1977), the sharp decrease in CML at age 0 (based on only 5 cases) may be explained by a shift towards diagnosing JMML/CMML at this age. On the other hand, a diagnostic group might combine disease subcategories that have different age distributions and different real time trends. For example, the rate of increase in total leukaemia was apparently slightly higher in infants (age group 0) than in older children. Although the difference was not statistically significant for total leukaemia, it was significant for AML, and it continued into recent years. It is possible that leukaemia in babies has been slightly under-reported or under-diagnosed until very recently, but it is also possible that there may have been a small real increase specific to that age group. Most cases of both ALL and AML in infants are associated with a chromosomal translocation involving the MLL gene (Biondi *et al.*, 2000); perhaps there has been a change in the risk of this occurring.

Similar arguments apply to differences in trend between boys and girls. For example, a likely explanation of the faster increase in girls than boys for CNS tumours overall is the relatively large increase in recorded incidence of astrocytoma, because the proportion of girls is higher in children with astrocytoma than with CNS tumours in general. On the other hand, the sex difference in the Hodgkin lymphoma trend might represent a real increase in the nodular sclerosing subtype, which has a higher-than-average proportion of girls (see Section 3.3) – this pattern was observed in the MCTR study (McNally *et al.*, 2001a).

A change in the underlying risk is the most interesting potential contributor to trends in recorded incidence rates. Little is definitely known about the causes of most childhood cancer, and separating real incidence trends from artefact is not easy, but the differences between diagnostic groups are large enough to suggest that, for some groups at least, there have been changes in risk. For example, the difference in trend between ALL and AML is probably mainly real. In childhood, both are acute diseases that are rapidly fatal without appropriate treatment. Diagnostic methods for leukaemia have been well established for many years, and the difference in trend is still evident in the most recent data (Fig. 4.1). It therefore seems likely that there has been a real increase in the risk of childhood ALL (Kroll *et al.*, 2006). For different reasons, the increase in malignant melanoma reported here is likely to be mainly real, in spite of the difficulties of diagnosis and coding described in Chapter 3. Similar trends have been reported in many settings for both children and adults, for example (McNally *et al.*, 2001b; Newnham and Møller, 2002; Pearce *et al.*, 2003; Ries *et al.*, 2006), and there is a plausible explanation – increasing exposure to sunlight.

In general, these increases in childhood cancer rates are quite small and fairly constant over time. There is no sign of any very large temporal change like those that have been associated with specific exogenous risk factors in other parts of the world, for example: the increase in Kaposi's sarcoma associated with the HIV epidemic in parts of Africa (Wabinga *et al.*, 2000); the apparently non-permanent increase in thyroid carcinoma in areas most heavily affected by radioactive deposition from Chernobyl (Antonelli *et al.*, 1996; Shibata *et al.*, 2001); the decrease in hepatocellular carcinoma following the introduction of Hepatitis-B immunization, which has been seen in Taiwan (Chang *et al.*, 1997) and is expected to follow in other countries. Any effects of environmental factors on incidence trends in Britain must be relatively subtle.

4.4 **Conclusion**

In this analysis, the recorded incidence of all childhood cancers together increased by slightly less than 1% per year on average over the 35-year study period, equivalent to a total increase of 38% from 1966 to 2000. The rate of increase ranged from 0.5 to 2.5% per year for the main diagnostic groups of ICCC-3, and varied widely between subgroups. These increases in recorded incidence do not necessarily represent real changes in risk, and it is important not to assume that they can all be explained by changes in some environmental carcinogen. Future trends will be monitored, and the trends will be analysed for possible contributing factors.

Chapter 5

Survival from Childhood Cancer

CA Stiller, ME Kroll and EM Eatock

This chapter presents the results of two sets of survival analyses. Details of the methodology can be found in Chapter 2.

The first part of this chapter consists of a detailed account of survival rates for children diagnosed with cancer in Britain during 1991–2000. The patients are the same as those on whom the incidence analyses given in Chapter 3 are based, except that children ascertained from a death certificate only or for whom no follow-up information was available have been excluded. More details of these exclusions can be found in Chapter 2. Survival rates are presented for all cancers combined and for the diagnostic groups, subgroups and divisions of ICCC-3. As in Chapter 3, results are also presented for subdivisions by immunophenotype, FAB classification, histological subtype, primary site and laterality. Unlike in Chapter 3, however, all non-Hodgkin lymphomas (NHL), including Burkitt lymphoma, are considered as a single diagnostic subgroup, within which Burkitt lymphoma constitutes one division rather than being regarded as a diagnostic subgroup in its own right. Variation in survival by sex and age was analysed for all groups, subgroups, divisions and subdivisions. Results are given separately for boys and girls or by age group only where the differences were statistically significant according to the log rank test.

The second set of analyses attempts to document the trends in survival for children diagnosed during 1966–2000. Results covering the full 35-year period are presented for all cancers combined and for the 12 diagnostic groups of ICCC-3. For ICCC-3 subgroups, divisions and selected subdivisions, the results generally relate to children diagnosed during 1971–2000. For some of these analyses, however, the starting date was later than 1971, because changes in the calculated incidence rates suggested that the composition of the relevant diagnostic category may have changed markedly within the study period. Changes in survival between calendar periods are expressed both as the simple arithmetic increase or decrease in percentage points and as the proportional increase or decrease in risk of death. For example, between 1966–70 and 1971–75 the 30-year survival rate for all cancers combined rose from 21.85 to 31.64%, an increase of 9.8 percentage points; the risk of death within 30 years of diagnosis decreased by $(78.15 - 68.36)/78.15 = 0.125$, or 12.5%.

The results of both sets of analyses are discussed in relation to other studies. Population-based analyses of childhood cancer survival across Europe have been published from two large international collaborations, namely EUROCARE (Capocaccia, Gatta, Magnani, Stiller, Coebergh, (Editors) 2001; Gatta *et al.*, 2003, 2005) and the

Automated Childhood Cancer Information System (ACCIS) (Steliarova-Foucher *et al.*, 2004, 2006a; Sankila *et al.*, 2006). The Surveillance, Epidemiology and End Results (SEER) Program *Pediatric Cancer Monograph* (Ries *et al.*, 1999) contains extensive analyses of childhood cancer survival in the USA. Reference is also made to other population-based studies that present survival rates based on reasonably large numbers of children. In discussing the effects of prognostic factors during the most recent decade, we also consider relevant results from large clinical trials and other non-population-based studies. Trends in survival are, where possible, related to the progress made in successive clinical trials that included substantial numbers of UK patients.

5.1 Survival of children diagnosed during 1991–2000

Table 5.1 gives numbers of children and actuarial survival rates at 1, 3, 5 and 10 years after diagnosis for all cancers combined and for diagnostic groups, subgroups and divisions with at least 20 cases diagnosed during 1991–2000 for whom follow-up was available. Some diagnostic subgroups and divisions had fewer than 20 registrations with follow-up from the period 1991–2000. For these rare diagnostic categories, the calendar period of diagnosis was extended backwards by one or more quinquennia in order to accrue sufficient cases for analysis. The results are shown in Table 5.2.

Overall survival was 88% at 1 year after diagnosis, 78% at 3 years, 75% at 5 years and 71% at 10 years. There was wide variation in survival between diagnostic groups, subgroups and divisions (Table 5.1 and Table 5.2). Among the 12 diagnostic groups in ICCC-3, ten-year survival ranged from 96% for retinoblastoma down to 55% for bone tumours and 53% for neuroblastoma and other peripheral nervous cell tumours. Survival varied more widely between ICCC-3 subgroups and divisions. Among subgroups, the highest ten-year survival was 100% for thyroid carcinoma, and the lowest was 20% for hepatic carcinoma. The lowest ten-year survival for any division was 0% for ATRT. Diagnostic categories with quite similar ten-year survival did not necessarily have similar risks of death throughout the 10 years since diagnosis. For example (Fig. 5.1), neuroblastoma, etc., and bone tumours had almost identical ten-year survival rates but the probability of dying during the first year following diagnosis was much higher for neuroblastoma, etc., 17%, than for bone tumours, 9%. In contrast, among children who survived 5 years from diagnosis, the probability of death during the next 5 years was only 4% for neuroblastoma, etc., but 11% for bone tumours. Among all the ICCC-3 subgroups and divisions included in Table 5.1, the highest probability of death by 3 years after diagnosis among those who had survived 1 year was 46% for (non-medulloblastoma) PNET. Among 3 year survivors, the highest probability of death by 5 years was 14% for CML and pPNET of soft tissue, and, among five-year survivors, the highest probability of death by 10 years was 27% for pPNET of bone.

For all cancers combined, five-year survival was slightly higher among girls (75%) than boys (74%), but the difference between the survival curves was not statistically significant. There was significant heterogeneity between the survival curves of children aged 0, 1–4, 5–9 and 10–14 years at diagnosis (log rank $p < 0.0001$). Five-year survival rates for

Text starts on page 139

Table 5.1 Survival of children with cancer diagnosed during 1991–2000. Numbers of children analysed (N) and actuarial survival rates at 1, 3, 5 and 10 years since diagnosis

Diagnostic groups	N	Survival (%) at time since diagnosis			
		1 year	3 years	5 years	10 years
All cancers	**14639**	**88**	**78**	**75**	**71**
Leukaemias, myeloproliferative and myelodysplastic diseases	**4691**	**91**	**81**	**77**	**73**
Lymphoid leukaemias	3715	95	87	82	77
Precursor cell leukaemias	3659	95	87	82	77
Mature B-cell leukaemias	54	76	74	74	72
Acute myeloid leukaemias	691	75	60	58	56
Chronic myeloid leukaemia	63	89	69	60	54
Myelodysplastic syndrome and other myeloproliferative diseases	173	76	56	51	49
Unspecified and other specified leukaemias	49	71	67	65	65
Lymphomas and reticuloendothelial neoplasms	**1423**	**91**	**87**	**86**	**84**
Hodgkin lymphomas	584	99	97	95	94
Non-Hodgkin lymphomas (including Burkitt lymphoma)	815	86	80	79	77
CNS and miscellaneous intracranial and intraspinal neoplasms	**3594**	**81**	**72**	**69**	**66**
Ependymomas and choroid plexus tumour	352	85	72	65	59
Ependymomas	261	90	75	66	59
Choroid plexus tumour	91	71	63	63	60
Astrocytomas	1550	86	80	79	76

Table 5.1 (continued) Survival of children with cancer diagnosed during 1991–2000. Numbers of children analysed (N) and actuarial survival rates at 1, 3, 5 and 10 years since diagnosis

Diagnostic groups	N	Survival (%) at time since diagnosis			
		1 year	3 years	5 years	10 years
Intracranial and intraspinal embryonal tumours	697	74	55	50	45
Medulloblastomas	509	81	64	58	53
Primitive neuroectodermal tumour (PNET)	161	56	30	27	23
Atypical teratoid/rhabdoid tumour	24	50	25	25	0
Other gliomas	379	60	44	42	39
Oligodendrogliomas	32	81	75	72	69
Mixed and unspecified gliomas	342	58	41	39	37
Other specified intracranial and intraspinal neoplasms	451	96	92	90	86
Pituitary adenomas and carcinomas	23	95	95	95	84
Tumours of the sellar region (craniopharyngiomas)	200	97	95	94	89
Pineal parenchymal tumours	38	84	63	55	52
Neuronal and mixed neuronal-glial tumours	142	96	94	94	91
Meningiomas	48	98	92	90	88
Unspecified intracranial and intraspinal neoplasms	165	72	71	71	69
Neuroblastoma and other peripheral nervous cell tumours	**896**	**83**	**61**	**56**	**53**
Neuroblastoma and ganglioneuroblastoma	885	83	60	55	53
Retinoblastoma	**430**	**99**	**97**	**96**	**96**
Renal tumours	**811**	**92**	**84**	**83**	**82**
Nephroblastoma and other nonepithelial renal tumours	787	92	85	83	82
Nephroblastoma	732	94	87	86	85

	N				
Rhabdoid renal tumour	24	38	25	25	25
Clear cell sarcoma of kidney	24	96	75	75	75
Hepatic tumours	**138**	**78**	**66**	**65**	**63**
Hepatoblastoma	112	83	76	75	72
Hepatic carcinomas	25	52	20	20	20
Malignant bone tumours	**563**	**91**	**68**	**62**	**55**
Osteosarcomas	307	88	64	57	50
Ewing tumour and related bone sarcomas	217	94	70	65	57
Soft tissue and other extraosseous sarcomas	**1027**	**87**	**70**	**65**	**62**
Rhabdomyosarcomas	547	89	69	66	64
Fibrosarcomas, peripheral nerve sheath tumours and other fibrous neoplasms	79	86	75	71	71
Fibroblastic and myofibroblastic tumours	37	86	84	84	84
Nerve sheath tumours	40	85	65	58	58
Other specified soft tissue sarcomas	340	86	73	66	61
Ewing tumour and Askin tumour of soft tissue	29	93	69	69	69
Peripheral neuroectodermal tumour (pPNET) of soft tissue	122	80	59	51	45
Fibrohistiocytic tumours	47	98	98	96	96
Synovial sarcomas	58	98	95	84	76
Unspecified soft tissue sarcomas	56	70	50	45	42
Germ cell tumours, trophoblastic tumours and neoplasms of gonads	**485**	**93**	**89**	**86**	**85**
Intracranial and intraspinal germ cell tumours	164	90	84	79	75
Intracranial and intraspinal germinomas	87	95	89	84	80

Table 5.1 (continued) Survival of children with cancer diagnosed during 1991–2000. Numbers of children analysed (N) and actuarial survival rates at 1, 3, 5 and 10 years since diagnosis

Diagnostic groups	N	Survival (%) at time since diagnosis			
		1 year	3 years	5 years	10 years
Intracranial and intraspinal teratomas	57	86	82	75	74
Malignant extracranial and extragonadal germ cell tumours	107	88	80	79	79
Malignant teratomas of extracranial and extragonadal sites	44	82	75	75	75
Yolk sac tumour of extracranial and extragonadal sites	54	96	87	85	85
Malignant gonadal germ cell tumours	204	99	97	96	96
Malignant gonadal germinomas	32	100	97	97	97
Malignant gonadal teratomas	75	97	96	93	93
Gonadal yolk sac tumour	82	100	99	99	99
Other malignant epithelial neoplasms and malignant melanomas	**482**	**93**	**88**	**86**	**85**
Adrenocortical carcinomas	24	83	54	50	50
Thyroid carcinomas	71	100	100	100	100
Nasopharyngeal carcinomas	24	100	83	83	83
Malignant melanomas	153	91	91	88	86
Skin carcinomas	82	99	99	99	93
Other and unspecified carcinomas	128	88	78	76	76
Carcinomas of salivary glands	30	100	97	97	97
Carcinomas of other specified sites	39	87	79	79	79
Other and unspecified malignant neoplasms	**99**	**95**	**91**	**90**	**90**
Other unspecified malignant tumours	82	96	96	95	95

Table 5.2 Survival of children with rare cancers diagnosed up to 2000. Calendar period of diagnosis, numbers of children analysed (N) and actuarial survival rates at 1, 3, 5 and 10 years since diagnosis

Diagnostic group	Years of diagnosis	N	Survival (%) at time since diagnosis			
			1 year	3 years	5 years	10 years
Lymphomas and reticuloendothelial neoplasms						
Miscellaneous lymphoreticular neoplasms	1981–2000	25	44	40	40	36
Unspecified lymphomas	1986–2000	26	80	80	76	76
Neuroblastoma and other peripheral nervous cell tumours						
Other peripheral nervous cell tumours	1981–2000	27	85	70	59	55
Renal tumours						
Renal carcinomas	1986–2000	23	83	83	83	83
Malignant bone tumours						
Chondrosarcomas	1981–2000	24	88	71	63	58
Other specified malignant bone tumours	1986–2000	28	89	82	82	82
Malignant fibrous neoplasms of bone	1971–2000	26	81	54	46	46
Unspecified malignant bone tumours	1981–2000	20	95	85	75	75
Soft tissue and other extraosseous sarcomas						
Other specified soft tissue sarcomas						
Extrarenal rhabdoid tumour	1986–2000	27	30	19	15	15
Liposarcomas	1971–2000	24	88	83	83	83
Leiomyosarcomas	1981–2000	26	100	88	85	81
Blood vessel tumours	1976–2000	25	72	68	52	52
Miscellaneous soft tissue sarcomas	1986–2000	22	86	55	50	50

Table 5.2 (continued) Survival of children with rare cancers diagnosed up to 2000. Calendar period of diagnosis, numbers of children analysed (N) and actuarial survival rates at 1, 3, 5 and 10 years since diagnosis

Diagnostic group	Years of diagnosis	N	Survival (%) at time since diagnosis			
			1 year	3 years	5 years	10 years
Germ cell tumours, trophoblastic tumours and neoplasms of gonads						
Malignant gonadal germ cell tumours						
Malignant gonadal tumours of mixed forms	1986–2000	20	95	90	90	90
Gonadal carcinomas	1986–2000	22	95	86	82	82
Other malignant epithelial neoplasms and malignant melanomas						
Other and unspecified carcinomas						
Carcinomas of colon and rectum	1981–2000	21	67	33	29	24
Carcinomas of appendix	1981–2000	21	100	100	95	95
Carcinomas of lung	1981–2000	21	95	95	95	95
Carcinomas of unspecified site	1981–2000	30	60	43	43	40
Other and unspecified malignant neoplasms						
Other specified malignant tumours	1981–2000	24	88	71	63	58

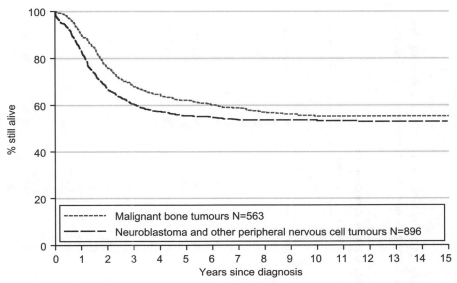

Fig. 5.1 Actuarial survival curves for children aged 0–14 years at diagnosis with neuroblastoma and other peripheral nervous cell tumours and malignant bone tumours. Great Britain, 1991–2000.

the age groups were 69, 76, 75 and 74%, respectively. The inferior prognosis for infants was entirely due to the much higher risk of death within 1 year after diagnosis, 22% compared with 11% for older children. Among one-year survivors, the risk of death during the next 4 years was in fact lower for infants than for older children. Table 5.3 shows survival by sex and age at diagnosis for diagnostic categories with at least 50 children followed up where there was significant variation between the sexes or between age groups. Survival differed significantly between boys and girls for lymphoid leukaemia, particularly precursor-cell ALL, neuroblastoma and malignant melanoma. In all of these categories, boys had lower survival than girls, and the gap tended to widen with increasing time since diagnosis.

Survival varied with age at diagnosis in a larger number of diagnostic categories. There were several patterns of age-related survival. For acute leukaemias, children in the middle-age range had higher survival than infants or children diagnosed at 10–14 years of age. For many types of CNS tumour, survival was higher for older children than for those diagnosed at a younger age. For neuroblastoma, infants had very much higher survival than children diagnosed after the first birthday. Children aged 10–14 years at diagnosis with Hodgkin lymphoma and rhabdomyosarcoma had a poorer prognosis than younger children.

The overall five-year survival of 74% for all cancers diagnosed during 1991–2000 was similar to the 75% observed for Western Europe during 1990–99 (Steliarova-Foucher *et al.*, 2004), and slightly higher than the 71% in the British Isles for children diagnosed predominantly during 1988–95 (Sankila *et al.*, 2006). Table 5.4 shows five-year survival rates in other large population-based studies of children diagnosed mainly in the 1990s. Survival in Britain from all cancers combined was comparable with that in Europe.

Text starts on page 146

Table 5.3 Variation in survival of children with cancer diagnosed during 1991–2000 by sex and age at diagnosis. Numbers of children analysed (N), actuarial survival rates at 1, 3, 5 and 10 years since diagnosis, and P-value from log rank test for heterogeneity of survival curves between boys and girls or between age groups

Diagnostic groups	Category	N	Survival (%) at time since diagnosis				P
			1 year	3 years	5 years	10 years	
Leukaemias, myeloproliferative and myelodysplastic diseases							
Lymphoid leukaemia	Boys	2107	94	86	81	76	0.0084
	Girls	1608	95	88	83	80	
	Age 0	128	73	50	44	39	<0.0001
	1–4	1944	97	92	88	84	
	5–9	1041	96	87	82	77	
	10–14	602	91	79	71	65	
Precursor cell ALL	Boys	2063	95	87	81	76	0.0097
	Girls	1596	95	88	83	80	
	Age 0	126	73	49	43	39	<0.0001
	1–4	1924	97	92	88	84	
	5–9	1024	96	88	83	77	
	10–14	585	91	79	70	65	
AML	Age 0	94	63	55	54	54	0.0179
	1–4	231	79	66	63	61	
	5–9	161	82	65	63	60	
	10–14	205	71	53	50	48	
Lymphomas and reticuloendothelial neoplasms							
Hodgkin lymphomas	Age 1–4	39	97	97	97	97	0.0121
	5–9	153	100	99	99	98	
	10–14	392	99	96	93	92	

	Age						p
Mature B-NHL (except Burkitt)	Age 1–9	35	77	71	71	71	0.0060
	10–14	53	98	94	94	92	
CNS and miscellaneous intracranial and intraspinal Neoplasms							
Ependymomas and choroid plexus tumours	Age 0	49	71	57	55	55	0.0037
	1–4	161	83	68	59	50	
	5–9	82	90	80	71	69	
	10–14	60	97	85	83	73	
Ependymomas	Age 0–4	134	87	69	58	48	0.0045
	5–9	71	89	79	68	68	
	10–14	56	98	86	84	73	
Astrocytomas	Age 0	74	78	70	64	55	<0.0001
	1–4	439	90	87	84	83	
	5–9	579	86	78	77	75	
	10–14	458	84	78	77	74	
Embryonal CNS	Age 0	64	28	19	17	17	<0.0001
	1–4	235	65	41	38	37	
	5–9	266	85	68	60	53	
	10–14	132	89	69	67	58	
Medulloblastoma	Age 0	29	48	34	34	34	<0.0001
	1–4	156	69	51	47	47	
	5–9	221	88	71	63	56	
	10–14	103	91	75	73	65	
PNET	Age 0	27	15	7	4	0	<0.0001
	1–4	68	56	19	18	14	
	5–9	40	68	53	48	42	
	10–14	26	81	50	46	33	

Table 5.3 (continued) Variation in survival of children with cancer diagnosed during 1991–2000 by sex and age at diagnosis. Numbers of children analysed (N), actuarial survival rates at 1, 3, 5 and 10 years since diagnosis, and P-value from log rank test for heterogeneity of survival curves between boys and girls or between age groups

Diagnostic groups	Category	N	Survival (%) at time since diagnosis				P
			1 year	3 years	5 years	10 years	
Other gliomas	Age 0–4	107	66	45	42	41	0.0026
	5–9	165	47	38	36	31	
	10–14	107	75	51	50	50	
Mixed/unspecified gliomas	Age 0–4	98	65	43	41	40	0.0122
	5–9	157	46	36	34	30	
	10–14	87	72	47	46	46	
Other specified CNS	Age 0	27	78	74	67	55	<0.0001
	1–4	81	96	84	83	79	
	5–9	158	96	94	91	87	
	10–14	185	98	96	96	93	
Unspecified CNS	Age 0–4	57	56	56	56	56	0.0001
	5–9	50	67	63	63	58	
	10–14	58	91	91	91	91	
Neuroblastoma and other peripheral nervous cell tumours							
Neuroblastoma	Boys	498	82	57	52	50	0.0360
	Girls	387	85	64	59	57	
	Age 0	257	89	84	83	83	<0.0001
	1–4	504	79	50	46	43	
	5–14	124	87	52	37	34	

Soft tissue and other extraosseous sarcomas

							p-value
Rhabdomyosarcoma	Age 0	47	87	70	66	66	0.0004
	1–4	248	91	70	67	65	
	5–9	170	90	75	72	71	
	10–14	82	84	54	48	45	
Other specified soft tissue sarcomas	Age 0	32	38	38	31	31	<0.0001
	1–4	58	86	76	69	65	
	5–9	91	91	78	70	68	
	10–14	159	92	75	69	62	

Germ cell tumours, trophoblastic tumours and neoplasms of gonads

							p-value
CNS germ-cell	Age 0–4	31	71	65	61	58	0.0032
	5–9	42	95	90	88	88	
	10–14	91	95	88	80	75	

Other malignant epithelial neoplasms and malignant melanomas

							p-value
Malignant melanoma	Boys	65	89	88	83	77	0.0094
	Girls	88	93	93	92	92	

Table 5.4 International comparison of survival of children with cancer diagnosed mainly in the 1990s. All results are five-year percentage survival

Cancer type	Great Britain[1] 1991–2000	Europe[1] 1990–94	Europe[1] 1988–97	United States[2] 1989–91	United States[2] 1995–2000	Japan[2] 1985–94
All cancers	74		72	73[3]	79[3]	68
Leukaemia	77		73			
ALL	82	79	79	80	85	60
AML	58	48	49	36	53	68
Lymphoma	85		84			67
Hodgkin lymphoma	95	94	93	94	96	
NHL	79	79[4]	77[5]	75	85	66
CNS	69		64	62[3]	73[3]	68
Ependymoma, etc.	66	55	58			
Astrocytoma	79	79	75			
PNET	50	50	49			
Sympathetic	56		59			75
Neuroblastoma	55	62	59	68	66	75
Retinoblastoma	96	91	93			93

	Great Britain (observed)	Great Britain (relative)	Europe EUROCARE	Europe ACCIS	United States SEER	Japan
Renal	83		84			75
Wilms', etc.	83	84	83	93	92	
Bone	62		61			
Osteosarcoma	57	66	59	62	73	
Ewing sarcoma	65	69	62			57
Soft tissue	65		65	78	75	
Rhabdomyosarcoma	66	67	63			63

[1] Observed survival

[2] Relative survival

[3] Excluding non-malignant CNS tumours

[4] Excluding Burkitt lymphoma

[5] Including miscellaneous and unspecified lymphomas

Sources: Great Britain, NRCT

Europe 1990–1994, EUROCARE (Gatta et al., 2003)

Europe 1988–1997, ACCIS (Clavel et al., 2006; Coebergh et al., 2006; Pastore et al., 2006a, 2006b; Peris-Bonet et al., 2006; Sankila et al., 2006; Spix et al., 2006; Stiller et al., 2006a)

United States, SEER (Jemal et al., 2005)

Japan, Osaka Cancer Registry (Ajiki et al., 2004)

The SEER registries of the USA reported slightly higher survival. The survival rates for Osaka, Japan, were lower, but this reflects the fact that the patients were diagnosed, on average, 6 years earlier than those in our study. International comparisons for specific diagnostic categories are discussed in succeeding sections of this chapter.

The small survival advantage of girls compared to boys has also been observed in the ACCIS study (Sankila *et al.*, 2006) and in New Zealand (Douglas and Dockerty, 2005). In Europe, five-year survival was slightly lower among infants than older children and, as in the present study, a higher proportion of deaths among infants occurred within the first year after diagnosis (Sankila *et al.*, 2006).

5.1.1 Leukaemias, myeloproliferative and myelodysplastic diseases

Overall, the ten-year survival rate for children in this group was 73%. The largest sub-group, lymphoid leukaemia, had a slightly higher ten-year survival of 77%. The sub-group consisted largely of precursor-cell ALL, also with ten-year survival of 77%. Among children with precursor-cell ALL of known immunophenotype, survival was highest for those with CD10-positive disease, intermediate for T-cell and lowest for null-cell (Fig. 5.2 and Table 5.5). Survival of children with no record of immunophenotype was similar to that of all children combined. Children with null-cell ALL had a higher chance of dying than those with CD10-positive ALL during each interval between diagnosis and 10 years later. The lower survival rate for T-cell ALL compared with CD10-positive was largely due to a much higher risk of death within 3 years after diagnosis. Boys with precursor-cell ALL fared less well than girls (Table 5.3). This applied particularly to CD10-positive leukaemia (Table 5.5); survival did not vary significantly by sex for the other

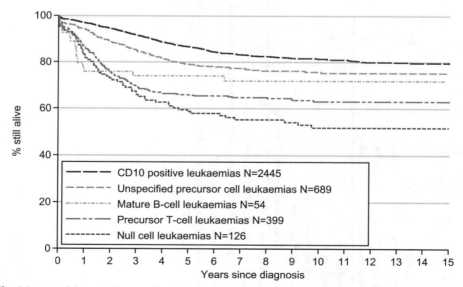

Fig. 5.2 Actuarial survival curves for children aged 0–14 years at diagnosis with precursor cell and mature B-cell leukaemias. Great Britain, 1991–2000.

Table 5.5 Survival of children with precursor-cell ALL diagnosed during 1991–2000 by immunophenotype. Numbers of children analysed (N) and actuarial survival rates at 1, 3, 5 and 10 years since diagnosis

Immunophenotype	N	Survival (%) at time since diagnosis			
		1 year	3 years	5 years	10 years
CD10 positive	2445	97	92	87	81
Boys	1366	97	92	85	79
Girls	1079	97	92	88	85
Age 0	32	72	56	53	50
1–4	1453	98	94	90	86
5–9	639	98	92	87	81
10–14	321	93	81	73	65
Null cell	126	83	67	59	52
Boys	67	88	69	63	60
Girls	59	78	64	54	44
Age 0	52	71	48	38	32
1–4	24	96	79	75	65
5–9	27	93	89	81	72
10–14	23	87	70	61	61
T-cell	399	86	70	66	63
Boys	263	85	69	66	62
Girls	136	89	71	66	64
Age 0–4	119	83	66	62	58
5–9	170	90	70	68	64
10–14	110	85	73	67	67
Other and unspecified	689	94	85	79	76
Boys	367	95	84	79	75
Girls	322	94	86	80	76
Age 0	36	75	49	46	46
1–4	334	96	90	86	83
5–9	188	95	87	81	76
10–14	131	93	81	68	65

immunophenotypes. Survival was highest for children with precursor-cell ALL diagnosed at 1–4 years of age, corresponding to the early childhood incidence peak, and declined with increasing age thereafter. Infants, however, were the age group with the lowest survival rate of all, 39% at 10 years. A similar effect of age was seen for CD10-positive and null cell leukaemia and for cases of unknown immunophenotype, but survival from T-cell ALL did not vary significantly with age. Children with mature B-cell leukaemia had slightly lower survival than those with precursor-cell ALL, but a much higher proportion of deaths occurred within 1 year of diagnosis (Fig. 5.2). The probability of death by 10 years from diagnosis among children who had survived 1 year was 18% for precursor-cell ALL and only 5% for mature B-cell leukaemia. Survival rates from mature B-cell leukaemia were similar for boys and girls.

Children with AML had lower survival than those with lymphoid leukaemia. As with precursor-cell ALL, infants and children aged 10–14 years had lower survival than children diagnosed at intermediate ages. However, the differences in survival rates between the age groups were less marked than for ALL, and survival was not so markedly inferior for infants. Indeed, infants with AML had higher survival than those with precursor-cell ALL (Fig. 5.3). A much higher proportion of deaths occurred within the first year after diagnosis for infants than for older children (Fig. 5.4). Survival did not differ significantly between boys and girls. Among children with known FAB subtype, survival was highest for M3 (promyelocytic) leukaemia (Table 5.6).

CML had a similar ten-year survival rate to AML, but mortality was lower than for AML during the first year after diagnosis and higher between 3 and 10 years after diagnosis (Fig. 5.5).

Myelodysplastic syndrome (MDS) and other myeloproliferative diseases formed the subgroup of leukaemias with the lowest survival (Fig. 5.5). Prognosis was especially poor for JMML/CMML (Table 5.7). Children with MDS had somewhat higher survival, similar to that for AML.

Children with unspecified or other specified leukaemia had a ten-year survival rate below that for all leukaemias combined but higher than that for any subgroup other than lymphoid leukaemia. Nearly all the deaths occurred within the first year after diagnosis. Within this subgroup, the 19 children with acute biphenotypic or mixed-lineage leukaemia had five-year survival of 79%, similar to that for precursor cell ALL.

Survival rates of children with leukaemia were similar to the European average in ACCIS, and survival rates for both ALL and AML were comparable with those achieved in most European regions (Coebergh *et al.*, 2006). Five-year survival rates for ALL and AML in France during 1990–2000 were identical to those in the present study

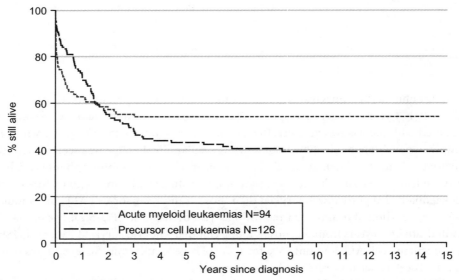

Fig. 5.3 Actuarial survival curves for infants aged under 1 year at diagnosis with acute leukaemia. Great Britain, 1991–2000.

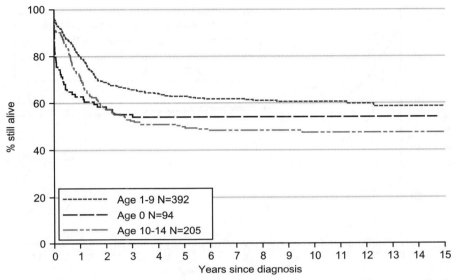

Fig. 5.4 Actuarial survival curves for children aged 0–14 years at diagnosis with acute myeloid leukaemia, by age at diagnosis. Great Britain, 1991–2000.

(Goubin *et al.*, 2006). Survival for both types of acute leukaemia was slightly higher in the Nordic countries (Gatta *et al.*, 2003; Coebergh *et al.*, 2006). Germany also had slightly higher survival for ALL, but not for AML (Gatta *et al.*, 2003). There are very few population-based data on outcome of mature B-cell leukaemia. Five-year survival in France during 1990–2000 was 85% (Goubin *et al.*, 2006), rather higher than in Britain.

Population-based series of childhood ALL have generally found a slightly better prognosis for girls than for boys, and a pattern of very poor survival among infants, with the highest survival among children diagnosed in the age range 1–4 years, and declining survival with increasing age thereafter (Smith *et al.*, 1999a; Stiller and Eatock, 1999;

Table 5.6 Survival of children with AML diagnosed during 1991–2000 by FAB type. Numbers of children analysed (N) and actuarial survival rates at 1, 3, 5 and 10 years since diagnosis

FAB type	N	Survival (%) at time since diagnosis			
		1 year	3 years	5 years	10 years
M1	53	83	55	55	52
M2	89	88	71	66	63
M3	59	83	71	71	66
M4	99	68	51	49	47
M5	118	64	59	57	55
M7	76	75	61	58	56
Other and unspecified	197	76	59	56	56

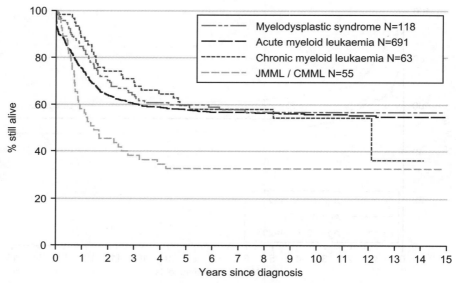

Fig. 5.5 Actuarial survival curves for children aged 0–14 years at diagnosis with non-lymphoid leukaemias and myelodysplastic syndrome. Great Britain, 1991–2000.

Viscomi *et al.*, 2003; Coebergh *et al.*, 2006; Goubin *et al.*, 2006). The difference in five-year survival between the sexes, often 2–4 percentage points, was much smaller than the differences of 7–10 percentage points in five-year event-free survival in many large European clinical trials (Conter *et al.*, 2000; Eden *et al.*, 2000; Schrappe *et al.*, 2000), suggesting that boys have a higher rate of occurrence of treatable relapse, though the Nordic countries provided an exception to this pattern (Gustafsson *et al.*, 2000). ALL of T-cell lineage always has a worse prognosis than precursor B-cell (Eden *et al.*, 2000; Gustafsson *et al.*, 2000; Goubin *et al.*, 2006). The markedly lower survival rate for null-cell ALL was similar to that in an earlier calendar period (Stiller and Eatock, 1999). Other important prognostic factors that were not analysed in the present study include white blood cell count, Down syndrome, CNS infiltration at diagnosis, and cytogenetics (Stiller and Eatock, 1999; Eden *et al.*, 2000).

In contrast to ALL, survival has not differed systematically between boys and girls with AML (Lie *et al.*, 2005; Goubin *et al.*, 2006). The relation between survival and age is also

Table 5.7 Survival of children with JMML/CMML and myelodysplastic syndrome diagnosed during 1991–2000. Numbers of children analysed (*N*) and actuarial survival rates at 1, 3, 5 and 10 years since diagnosis

Diagnosis	N	Survival (%) at time since diagnosis			
		1 year	3 years	5 years	10 years
JMML/CMML	55	58	38	33	33
Myelodysplastic syndrome	118	85	64	60	57

less clear-cut (Smith *et al.*, 1999a; Gibson *et al.*, 2005; Coebergh *et al.*, 2006). In particular, diagnosis in the first year of life was not an adverse factor. Within the UK national trials, as in this population-based study, infants with AML had higher survival than those with ALL (Chessells *et al.*, 2002a). The high survival rate for M3 AML was also found in contemporary national trials in the UK (Gibson *et al.*, 2005) and in population-based data from France (Goubin *et al.*, 2006). The favourable prognosis for the M3 subtype is also found among adults with AML (Hann *et al.*, 1997). In marked contrast to ALL, Down syndrome is not an adverse factor in AML, and children with Down syndrome have had higher survival than other children in recent studies (Lie *et al.*, 1996; Rao *et al.*, 2006).

We know of no previous population-based survival data for CML in children, as opposed to the combined group of CML and JMML/CMML. Survival rates for JMML/CMML and MDS were consistent with those reported from the UK paediatric MDS register for a slightly different calendar period (Passmore *et al.*, 2003).

5.1.2 Lymphomas and reticuloendothelial neoplasms

The ten-year survival rate for all lymphomas combined was 84%. Survival was highest for Hodgkin lymphomas, 94% at 10 years (Fig. 5.6). Age was a significant prognostic factor for Hodgkin lymphoma (Table 5.3), with lower survival among children diagnosed at age 10–14 years. The effect of age was least pronounced in the first year following diagnosis. Boys and girls had similar survival rates. Survival by histological subtype is shown in Table 5.8. Lymphocyte-rich classical and nodular-lymphocytic-predominant – both had

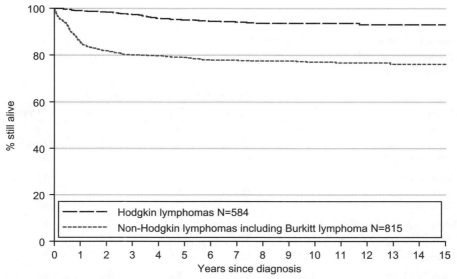

Fig. 5.6 Actuarial survival curves for children aged 0–14 years at diagnosis with Hodgkin and non-Hodgkin lymphomas. Great Britain, 1991–2000.

Table 5.8 Survival of children with non-Hodgkin lymphomas diagnosed during 1991–2000 by histological subtype. Numbers of children analysed (N) and actuarial survival rates at 1, 3, 5 and 10 years since diagnosis

Subtype	N	Survival (%) at time since diagnosis			
		1 year	3 years	5 years	10 years
Nodular lymphocyte predominant	49	100	100	100	100
Other lymphocyte-rich/predominant	44	100	100	100	100
Mixed cellularity	80	98	95	95	95
Nodular sclerosis	351	99	97	93	91
Other and unspecified	60	98	98	97	95

100% ten-year survival. Survival was slightly lower for the mixed-cellularity and nodular-sclerosing subtypes.

Non-Hodgkin lymphoma (NHL), including Burkitt lymphoma, had ten-year survival of 77% (Fig. 5.6), similar to that for lymphoid leukaemias. Table 5.9 and Fig. 5.7 show survival for NHL, categorized according to cell lineage and maturity. Among both precursor-cell and mature-cell NHL, children with T-cell disease had lower survival than those with B-cell. This was also true for NHL overall despite the anomaly of higher survival for T-cell than for B-cell among patients of unknown cell maturity. Age was not a significant prognostic factor for NHL as a whole, but among children with non-Burkitt mature B-cell lymphoma, those aged 10–14 years at diagnosis had significantly higher survival. This could well have been a chance finding, however, as there were no

Table 5.9 Survival of children with non-Hodgkin lymphomas diagnosed during 1991–2000 by histological subtype. Numbers of children analysed (N) and actuarial survival rates at 1, 3, 5 and 10 years since diagnosis

Subtype	N	Survival (%) at time since diagnosis			
		1 year	3 years	5 years	10 years
Precursor cell	174	90	78	75	69
Precursor B-cell	21	95	90	86	76
Precursor T-cell	153	89	76	73	68
Mature B-cell	279	87	84	84	82
Burkitt	191	86	83	83	81
Other mature B-cell	88	90	85	85	84
Mature T-cell and NK-cell	124	81	74	73	72
Anaplastic large-cell	90	81	74	74	74
Unspecified T-cell	49	90	84	82	82
Unspecified B-cell	138	83	81	81	80
Other unspecified	51	82	76	76	76

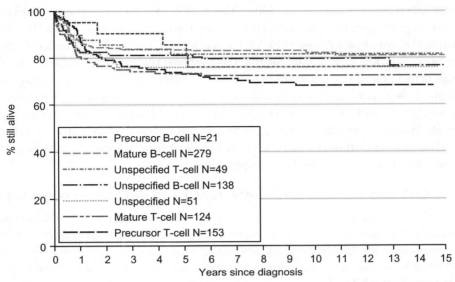

Fig. 5.7 Actuarial survival curves for children aged 0–14 years at diagnosis with non-Hodgkin lymphomas (including Burkitt lymphoma) by cell lineage and maturity. Great Britain, 1991–2000.

significant age effects for any other category of NHL, and for Burkitt lymphoma younger children had higher survival, though not significantly so. Overall, children aged 5–9 years at diagnosis with NHL in the multicentre BFM studies (which included patients aged 0–18 years) had higher event-free survival than younger or older patients (Burkhardt *et al.*, 2005); among children aged under 15 years, precursor B-cell NHL was the only category for which age was a significant prognostic factor, with those aged 0–4 years having the worst outcome.

Survival rates were lowest for the subgroup of miscellaneous lymphoreticular neoplasms, while unspecified lymphomas had similar survival to NHL. Each of these subgroups had fewer than 20 cases with follow-up diagnosed during 1991–2000, but results are shown in Table 5.2 for miscellaneous lymphoreticular neoplasms diagnosed in 1981–2000 and for unspecified lymphomas in 1986–2000. Nearly all the deaths in both subgroups occurred within 1 year of diagnosis.

The very high survival rate for children with Hodgkin lymphoma is typical of western industrialized countries (Percy *et al.*, 1999; Gatta *et al.*, 2003; Clavel *et al.*, 2006). The slightly lower survival in older children was also observed in ACCIS (Clavel *et al.*, 2006). In the UKCCSG's first Hodgkin's disease study, histological subtype had no effect on survival when disease stage was taken into account (Shankar *et al.*, 1997). In that study, stage III and IV accounted for 39% of nodular sclerosing cases, 31% of mixed cellularity cases and 17% of lymphocyte-predominant cases. It seems likely that the variation in survival with subtype in the present study also reflects differing distributions of stage by subtype.

Survival from NHL (including Burkitt lymphoma) was similar to that in the Nordic countries and Southern Europe but slightly lower than in the Western Europe region of the ACCIS study (Izarzugaza *et al.*, 2006). The EUROCARE study found higher survival in two large Western European countries, namely Germany and France, for NHL other than Burkitt lymphoma during 1990–94 (Gatta *et al.*, 2003). In the French national series for 1990–2000, five-year survival for all NHL combined was 87% (Goubin *et al.*, 2006). As in Britain, survival was lower for precursor T-cell NHL and close to the average for anaplastic large cell lymphoma. Results for B-cell NHL could not be reliably compared because of the markedly different relative frequencies of Burkitt and non-Burkitt lymphoma in the two countries (see also Chapter 3). It is notable, however, that the French survival rate for Burkitt lymphoma was exceptionally high, as was also observed for mature B-cell leukaemia, its leukaemic equivalent.

5.1.3 CNS and miscellaneous intracranial and intraspinal neoplasms

Overall ten-year survival for children with any type of CNS tumour was 66%. Survival varied considerably between subgroups and divisions within this large and very heterogeneous diagnostic group. Survival for ICCC-3 subgroups and divisions is shown in Table 5.1. Results for other pathological categories are shown in Table 5.10 and by primary site in Table 5.11.

Ependymomas and choroid plexus tumours had survival rates similar to the average for CNS tumours. For the subgroup as a whole and for ependymomas, survival was significantly lower for children diagnosed below age 5 years (Table 5.3). Among ependymomas, survival was especially high for spinal cord tumours, intermediate for supratentorial sites and lowest for cerebellar tumours (Table 5.11). Within the choroid plexus tumours, survival was high for papillomas and low for carcinomas, 94 and 17%, respectively, at 10 years (Table 5.10).

Survival of children with astrocytomas was higher than the average for CNS tumours. Survival was lowest for infants, highest for children aged 1–4 years and intermediate for

Table 5.10 Survival of children with selected CNS tumours diagnosed during 1991–2000 by pathological subtype. Numbers of children analysed (N) and actuarial survival rates at 1, 3, 5 and 10 years since diagnosis

Tumour type	N	\multicolumn{4}{c}{Survival (%) at time since diagnosis}			
		1 year	3 years	5 years	10 years
Choroid plexus tumours					
Papilloma	51	96	96	96	94
Carcinoma	40	40	20	20	17
Astrocytoma					
Grade 1–2	1179	96	94	92	89
Grade 3–4	238	43	19	17	16
Unspecified grade	133	73	68	68	67
Neuronal and mixed neuronal–glial tumours					
Ganglioglioma	69	93	91	90	87
Dysembryoplastic neuroepithelial tumour	62	100	100	100	98

Table 5.11 Survival of children with selected CNS tumours diagnosed during 1991–2000 by primary site. Numbers of children analysed (N) and actuarial survival rates at 1, 3, 5 and 10 years since diagnosis

Tumour type	N	Survival (%) at time since diagnosis			
		1 year	3 years	5 years	10 years
Ependymoma					
Supratentorial brain	47	96	83	72	64
Cerebellum	135	90	69	58	47
Other and unspecified brain	47	81	72	62	59
Spinal cord	30	97	97	97	97
Astrocytoma					
Supratentorial brain	389	78	65	63	59
Cerebellum	504	97	96	95	94
Brain stem	180	52	37	37	33
Ventricles	71	93	92	90	90
Other & unspecified brain	115	90	86	85	80
Optic nerve	214	99	97	94	94
Spinal cord	75	88	84	81	75
Mixed and unspecified gliomas					
Supratentorial brain	81	81	72	70	65
Brain stem	214	44	22	20	18
Other & unspecified CNS	47	83	74	72	72

those aged 5–14 years at diagnosis (Table 5.3). Grade was a highly important prognostic factor (Table 5.10). Survival rates at 10 years from diagnosis were 89% for grades 1–2 and 16% for grades 3–4. Survival also varied by primary site (Table 5.11). Astrocytomas of the cerebellum, ventricles and optic nerve all had ten-year survival of at least 90%. Survival was lower for spinal cord and supratentorial brain primaries and lowest of all, 33% at 10 years, for brain stem astrocytomas.

Embryonal CNS tumours had ten-year survival of 45%. For the subgroup as a whole and for the two main divisions of medulloblastoma and other PNET, survival was lower for children below 5 years of age and especially so for infants (Fig. 5.8 and Table 5.3). The effect of age was largely attributable to higher mortality among young children during the first few years after diagnosis. Ten-year survival was 53% for medulloblastoma but only 23% for other PNET, while there were no ten-year survivors with ATRT (Fig. 5.9). It has been suggested that misclassification of some cases of ATRT as medulloblastoma or other PNET might have exaggerated the poorer prognosis of younger children in these more numerous diagnostic categories (McNeil *et al.*, 2002).

Other gliomas had a low survival rate. This subgroup was dominated by the division of mixed and unspecified gliomas, which had similarly low survival. Unusually, survival was lower for children diagnosed at age 5–9 years than for younger or older children (Table 5.3). Prognosis varied markedly by site, with ten-year survival below 20% for brain stem tumours and above 60% for those in supratentorial sites (Table 5.11). The other division within this subgroup, oligodendrogliomas, had a ten-year survival rate of 69%.

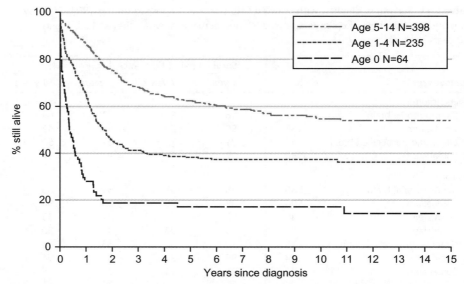

Fig. 5.8 Actuarial survival curves for children aged 0–14 years at diagnosis with intracranial and intraspinal embryonal tumours, by age at diagnosis. Great Britain, 1991–2000.

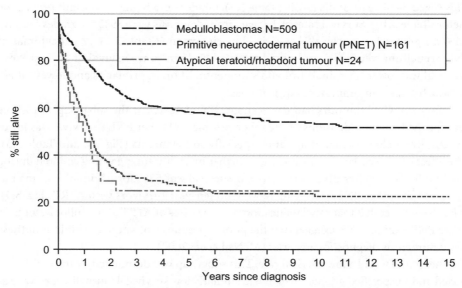

Fig. 5.9 Actuarial survival curves for children aged 0–14 years at diagnosis with intracranial and intraspinal embryonal tumours, by histological subtype. Great Britain, 1991–2000.

Overall, the miscellaneous subgroup of other specified CNS tumours had a ten-year survival rate of 86%. Survival was lower for infants than for children diagnosed after the first birthday (Table 5.3). Of the divisions within this subgroup, pituitary adenomas and carcinomas, craniopharyngioma, neuronal–glial tumours and meningiomas all had ten-year survival in excess of 80% (Tables 5.1 and 5.2). Within the neuronal–glial division, dysembryoplastic neuroepithelial tumours had an especially high survival rate (Table 5.9). Pineal parenchymal tumours had markedly lower survival, 52% at 10 years.

Unspecified CNS tumours had a 69% ten-year survival rate. Nearly all deaths occurred within 1 year after diagnosis. Survival increased with age at diagnosis (Table 5.3).

The overall five-year survival rate of 69% for CNS tumours was higher than the 63% for these tumours diagnosed in the British Isles during 1988–97, though still slightly below the 72% observed in the Nordic countries over the same period (Peris-Bonet *et al.*, 2006). The markedly lower survival of very young children, especially those with embryonal tumours or ependymoma, was similar to the pattern in Europe and the USA (Gurney *et al.*, 1999a; McNeil *et al.*, 2002; Peris-Bonet *et al.*, 2006). In Germany during 1990–99, survival rates were similar to those reported here for astrocytoma, medulloblastoma and craniopharyngioma, slightly lower (61%) for ependymoma and markedly higher for supratentorial PNET (47%) (Kaatsch *et al.*, 2001).

In Germany, as in Britain, low-grade astrocytoma had a much better prognosis than high-grade, with five-year survival rates of 85 and 27%, respectively. These survival rates should not be compared directly with those for Britain, however, since 8.6% of cases in the British series were of unspecified grade, compared with only 4.6% in Germany. Survival rates for astrocytoma, craniopharyngioma, ganglioglioma, meningioma and pineal parenchymal tumours were similar to the European average for 1988–97 (Peris-Bonet *et al.*, 2006). The markedly lower survival for supratentorial PNET compared to infratentorial, predominantly medulloblastoma, was also found in the USA (McNeil *et al.*, 2002).

5.1.4 Neuroblastoma and other peripheral nervous cell tumours

This group had the lowest ten-year survival of any ICCC-3 group, 53%. It was dominated by neuroblastoma, for which survival was almost identical. Neuroblastoma was one of the few subgroups for which survival differed significantly between the sexes (Table 5.3). Boys had lower survival than girls, and the gap widened with time since diagnosis. There was also a marked effect of age on survival (Fig. 5.10 and Table 5.3). Survival decreased with age at diagnosis, and the difference was especially pronounced between infants and children diagnosed at 1–4 years of age, with five-year survival of 83 and 43%, respectively. The effect of age also increased with time since diagnosis. Among one-year survivors, the probabilities of survival to 10 years for children aged under 1 year, 1–4 years and 5–14 years at diagnosis were 93, 54 and 39%, respectively. Primary site was also an important prognostic factor (Table 5.12). The sites fell into two groups with similar survival rates; 43–53% of children with adrenal, abdominal or unspecified primary site survived for 10 years, compared to 69–90% for the other site categories (Fig. 5.11).

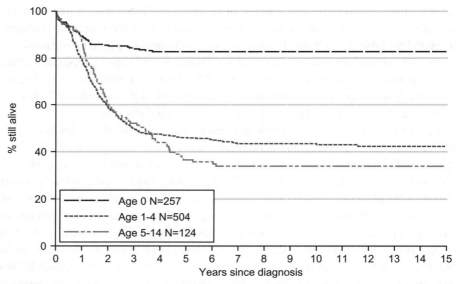

Fig. 5.10 Actuarial survival curves for children aged 0–14 years at diagnosis with neuroblastoma (including ganglioneuroblastoma), by age at diagnosis. Great Britain, 1991–2000.

There were too few cases of other sympathetic nervous system tumours diagnosed during 1991–2000 for analysis, but survival of those diagnosed during 1981–2000 was similar to that for neuroblastoma (Table 5.2).

The most important prognostic factors in neuroblastoma are age at diagnosis and stage (Breslow and McCann, 1971; Kinnier Wilson and Draper, 1974; Bernstein *et al.*, 1992; Cotterill *et al.*, 2000c). Infants have higher survival than older children. Children with localized tumours, or with stage 4S disease, which usually regresses spontaneously, have markedly higher survival than those with stage 4 disease at diagnosis. Older children with metastatic neuroblastoma have an especially poor prognosis. The lower survival for children with abdominal or unknown primary site presumably reflects their higher proportion of later-stage disease. In the European Neuroblastoma Study Group (ENSG) Survey, 69% of cases with abdominal primary site were stage 4, compared to 32% for other specified sites (Cotterill *et al.*, 2000c). There is wide international variation in the detection rate of asymptomatic neuroblastoma in infants, even in the absence of mass screening. As these tumours have an excellent prognosis, there is strong correlation between the incidence rate in the first year of life and the survival rate for children of all ages combined (Spix *et al.*, 2006). Consequently, international comparisons of survival from neuroblastoma are of limited value unless age is taken into consideration. Five-year survival of infants was very similar to that in Europe (Spix *et al.*, 2006) and the USA (Goodman *et al.*, 1999). Survival was lower than in the USA, however, for children aged 1–4 (Goodman *et al.*, 1999) and lower than in the USA and Europe for those aged 5 years and above (Goodman *et al.*, 1999; Spix *et al.*, 2006), despite the fact that children in the other two studies were diagnosed during a calendar period that was, on average, 3–5 years earlier.

Table 5.12 Survival of children with neuroblastoma and selected bone and soft tissue sarcomas diagnosed during 1991–2000 by primary site. Numbers of children analysed (N) and actuarial survival rates at 1, 3, 5 and 10 years since diagnosis

Tumour type	Survival (%) at time since diagnosis				
	N	1 year	3 years	5 years	10 years
Neuroblastoma					
Head and neck	28	89	82	79	79
Thoracic	115	97	87	84	83
Adrenal	408	80	53	47	45
Other abdominal	227	78	52	46	43
Pelvic	30	100	93	90	90
Other and unspecified trunk	23	96	78	74	69
Unspecified	54	81	59	55	53
Osteosarcoma					
Arm	37	86	70	67	51
Leg	254	89	64	57	51
Ewing's and related bone sarcomas					
Arm	25	96	72	60	55
Leg	94	96	77	72	64
Pelvis, etc.	50	88	53	49	42
Other specified	47	94	74	68	60
Rhabdomyosarcoma					
Orbit	51	98	90	86	86
Other head and neck	175	89	69	63	62
Bladder and prostate	54	100	91	87	83
Other genitourinary	75	100	97	95	93
Other trunk	126	82	51	48	48
Extremity	54	81	41	39	33
Synovial sarcoma					
Leg	31	97	90	84	80
Other specified	27	100	100	85	73

5.1.5 Retinoblastoma

Survival from retinoblastoma was high. There was little difference between the survival rates for unilateral and bilateral disease, with more than 90% of children in both groups surviving 10 years (Table 5.13).

The high survival rate for retinoblastoma was typical of western industrialized countries (Young *et al.*, 1999; MacCarthy *et al.*, 2006). Within 10 years of diagnosis, bilateral cases had only slightly lower survival than unilateral. The difference becomes more pronounced at longer intervals after diagnosis, principally because of the much higher risk of second malignancies among survivors of bilateral retinoblastoma (Draper *et al.*, 1986; Moll *et al.*, 1997).

5.1.6 Renal tumours

This group was dominated by nephroblastoma (Wilms' tumour). For the group as a whole and for nephroblastoma, ten-year survival was over 80%. Most deaths occurred

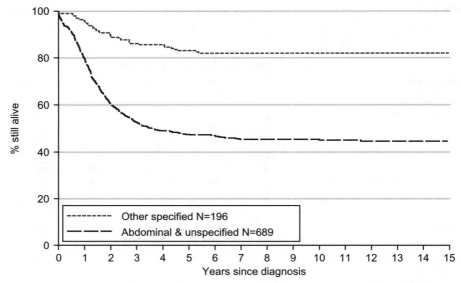

Fig. 5.11 Actuarial survival curves for children aged 0–14 years at diagnosis with neuroblastoma (including ganglioneuroblastoma), by primary site. Great Britain, 1991–2000.

within 3 years from diagnosis. The prognosis was poorer for children with bilateral tumours than for those with unilateral disease (Fig. 5.12 and Table 5.13), with the difference being most marked between 1 and 3 years after diagnosis.

Rhabdoid renal tumour had much lower survival, 25% at 10 years. Nearly two-thirds of children with this tumour died within a year of diagnosis. Survival from clear cell sarcoma of the kidney was somewhat lower than from nephroblastoma, 75% at 10 years. The difference only emerged beyond 1 year from diagnosis. There were fewer than 20 children with renal carcinoma diagnosed during 1991–2000, but ten-year survival of those diagnosed during 1986–2000 was 83%, comparable with outcome from nephroblastoma (Table 5.2).

Five-year survival from nephroblastoma was lower than in the USA (Bernstein *et al.*, 1999a), the Nordic countries and Western Europe, and comparable with Southern

Table 5.13 Survival of children with retinoblastoma and nephroblastoma diagnosed during 1991–2000 by laterality. Numbers of children analysed (N) and actuarial survival rates at 1, 3, 5 and 10 years since diagnosis

Tumour type	N	Survival (%) at time since diagnosis			
		1 year	3 years	5 years	10 years
Retinoblastoma					
Unilateral	272	99	97	96	96
Bilateral	151	99	97	95	94
Nephroblastoma					
Unilateral	661	94	88	87	86
Bilateral	52	92	77	73	73

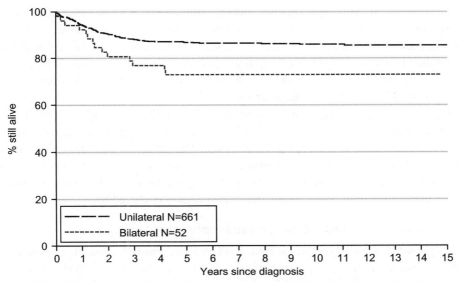

Fig. 5.12 Actuarial survival curves for children aged 0–14 years at diagnosis with nephroblastoma (Wilms' tumour), by laterality. Great Britain, 1991–2000.

Europe (Pastore *et al.*, 2006b). In Europe, survival was lower for children diagnosed at age 5 years and above (Pastore *et al.*, 2006b). In Britain, survival did not vary significantly with age at diagnosis, though the very few children diagnosed at age 10–14 had a somewhat lower five-year survival of 71%. Children with bilateral nephroblastoma had lower survival than unilateral in the USA and Europe (Bernstein *et al.*, 1999a; Pastore *et al.*, 2006b). Survival rates for rhabdoid renal tumour and clear cell sarcoma of the kidney were similar to those in Europe and the USA (Bernstein *et al.*, 1999a; Pastore *et al.*, 2006b). In the National Wilms' Tumor Study, older age at diagnosis was a favourable prognostic factor for rhabdoid renal tumour (Tomlinson *et al.*, 2005), but there was no sign of this in our data.

5.1.7 Hepatic tumours

Ten-year survival for hepatic tumours as a whole was 63%. Survival was much higher for hepatoblastoma (72% at 10 years) than for hepatic carcinoma (20%). Most deaths in both subgroups occurred within 3 years of diagnosis.

The relatively good prognosis for hepatoblastoma and the very poor survival for hepatic carcinoma have also been observed in Europe and the USA (Darbari *et al.*, 2003; Stiller *et al.*, 2006d).

5.1.8 Malignant bone tumours

Bone tumours were the ICCC-3 group with the second lowest ten-year survival, 55%. Of the two main subgroups, osteosarcoma had lower survival than Ewing tumour. There were too few cases of the other subgroups diagnosed during 1991–2000 for analysis.

When cases from earlier years were included, chondrosarcoma and malignant fibrous neoplasms appeared to have similar survival to the group as a whole (Table 5.2). Nearly all osteosarcomas occurred in the limbs, and survival was similar for children with primary site in the arm or leg (Table 5.12). Survival from Ewing tumour varied substantially by primary site (Table 5.12). Children with pelvic primaries had much lower survival than those with Ewing tumour of other sites.

Survival rates for osteosarcoma were lower than in the USA and most of Europe (Gurney *et al.*, 1999c; Stiller *et al.*, 2006a). For Ewing tumour, survival was comparable with that in the USA and Europe (Gurney *et al.*, 1999c; Stiller *et al.*, 2006a). As found in other studies, pelvic primary site was a poor prognostic factor for Ewing tumour (Gurney *et al.*, 1999c; Cotterill *et al.*, 2000a; Stiller *et al.*, 2006c), probably because of the larger tumour volume associated with that site (Cotterill *et al.*, 2000a).

5.1.9 Soft tissue and other extraosseous sarcomas

Ten-year survival for all soft tissue sarcomas combined was 62%. Rhabdomyosarcoma, which accounted for slightly over half of the group, had similar survival. Among the other subgroups and divisions with at least 20 cases diagnosed during 1991–2000, survival was especially high for fibrohistiocytic tumours and lowest for peripheral PNET. Among the rarer divisions of other specified soft tissue sarcomas for which longer periods had to be analysed, ten-year survival exceeded 80% for liposarcoma and leiomyosarcoma, but was only 15% for extrarenal rhabdoid tumour. Relatively low survival rates were also observed for blood vessel tumours and the heterogeneous category of miscellaneous specified sarcomas. More than half of the latter were desmoplastic small round cell tumour, for which the ten-year survival, based on 12 cases, was 25%.

Age was an important prognostic factor for rhabdomyosarcoma, children diagnosed at 10–14 years of age having a ten-year survival rate of under 50%, compared with at least 65% for younger children (Table 5.3). Survival also varied with age for the diverse subgroup of other specified soft tissue sarcomas; diagnosis during infancy was associated with a low survival rate. Among children with rhabdomyosarcoma, histological subtype was also of prognostic importance (Table 5.14). Alveolar histology had lower survival than embryonal, and the gap increased with time since diagnosis (Fig. 5.13). Survival from rhabdomyosarcoma varied according to primary site (Table 5.12). The highest

Table 5.14 Survival of children with rhabdomyosarcoma diagnosed during 1991–2000 by histological subtype. Numbers of children analysed (N) and actuarial survival rates at 1, 3, 5 and 10 years since diagnosis

| Tumour type | N | Survival (%) at time since diagnosis | | | |
		1 year	3 years	5 years	10 years
Embryonal	341	93	77	74	73
Alveolar	123	85	49	42	39
Unspecified	83	83	70	67	65

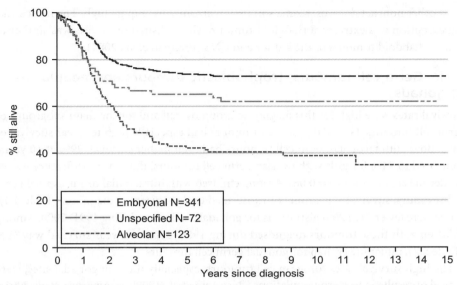

Fig. 5.13 Actuarial survival curves for children aged 0–14 years at diagnosis with rhabdomyosarcoma, by histological subtype. Great Britain, 1991–2000.

survival was for children with genitourinary or orbital tumours. Other head and neck sites had somewhat lower survival, followed by other sites in the trunk. The prognosis for rhabdomyosarcoma of the extremities was even worse, with only one-third of children surviving 10 years. In contrast, among children with synovial sarcoma, there was little difference in survival between tumours of the leg, the most frequent primary site, and those of other sites (Table 5.12).

Survival rates for soft tissue sarcomas overall and for rhabdomyosarcomas in particular were comparable with those in the USA and Europe (Gurney *et al.*, 1999e; Punyko *et al.*, 2005; Pastore *et al.*, 2006a). In common with other studies, children with rhabdomyosarcoma diagnosed at 10–14 years of age had lower survival than younger children (Joshi *et al.*, 2004; Punyko *et al.*, 2005; Pastore *et al.*, 2006a). In other European and American studies, infants also had a worse prognosis (Joshi *et al.*, 2004; Punyko *et al.*, 2005; Pastore *et al.*, 2006a), but in the present study they had a similar prognosis to children aged 1–4 years at diagnosis.

The pattern of survival from rhabdomyosarcoma by histological subtype and primary site was similar to that in the United States SEER registries and in the SIOP MMT-89 trial (Punyko *et al.*, 2005; Stevens *et al.*, 2005). We were unable to classify all head and neck primaries as parameningeal or not on the basis of ICD-O-3 topographical codes. Parameningeal tumours are regarded as having a worse prognosis, but in the SIOP study, while their event-free survival was lower than for nonparameningeal tumours, overall survival was identical for the two groups (Stevens *et al.*, 2005).

The prognosis for extraosseous Ewing sarcoma family tumours was similar to that for Ewing tumour of bone, as is also the case in adults (Verrill *et al.*, 1997). Survival rates for most other nonrhabdomyosarcoma soft tissue sarcomas were quite high. The most striking exception was extrarenal rhabdoid tumour, whose dismal prognosis was similar to that of rhabdoid tumours of the kidney and CNS (Brennan *et al.*, 2004).

5.1.10 Germ cell tumours, trophoblastic tumours and neoplasms of gonads

Survival rates were high for this diagnostic group overall and for the main subgroups of germ cell tumours. Gonadal germ cell tumours had especially high ten-year survival of 96%. Boys with testicular germ cell tumours had even higher survival, 99% at 10 years, compared to 94% for girls with ovarian germ cell tumours, though the difference was of borderline significance ($p = 0.06$). Among children with intracranial or intraspinal germ cell tumours, survival was lower for those aged under 5 years at diagnosis (Table 5.3). There were fewer than 20 registrations for gonadal carcinoma during 1991–2000. Among children with these tumours diagnosed during 1986–2000, ten-year survival was 82% (Table 5.2), rather lower than for gonadal germ cell tumours.

The high survival rates for germ cell tumours, especially those in gonadal sites, were typical of results in western populations (Bernstein *et al.*, 1999b; Kramarova *et al.*, 2001). Gonadal carcinomas had a somewhat lower survival rate than in the SEER registries but this is likely to be at least partly due to the exclusion of borderline tumours that have an excellent prognosis (Bernstein *et al.*, 1999b).

5.1.11 Other malignant epithelial neoplasms and malignant melanomas

There was substantial variation in survival between subgroups and divisions within this diagnostic group, with ten-year survival ranging from 100% for carcinomas of the thyroid and 97% for salivary gland carcinoma to 50% for adrenocortical carcinoma among children diagnosed during 1991–2000. There were too few children with adrenocortical carcinoma to be included in Table 5.3, but ten-year survival was markedly higher for the 15 children aged 0–4 years at diagnosis (73%) than for the nine aged 5–14 years (11%). No deaths have yet been observed among children with thyroid carcinoma of any histological subtype diagnosed during 1991–2000. Among those diagnosed during 1971–2000, however, 20-year survival was lower for medullary carcinoma (63%) than for differentiated carcinoma (99%). For carcinomas of the nasopharynx and skin, ten-year survival was above 80 and 90%, respectively. Among the rarer carcinomas with under 20 registrations during 1991–2000, the ten-year survival of children diagnosed during 1981–2000 was 95% for tumours of the appendix and lung, but only 40% for carcinoma of unspecified primary site and 24% for colorectal carcinoma (Table 5.2). There were only 14 children registered with bladder carcinoma throughout 1971–2000; no deaths have been recorded among them.

Malignant melanoma had ten-year survival of 86%. The prognosis was worse for boys than for girls (Table 5.3). Children with ocular malignant melanoma had a high survival rate (88% based on eight cases) but all nine children with CNS melanoma died less than 6 months after diagnosis.

Outcome for adrenocortical carcinoma was similar to that in EUROCARE (Gatta *et al.*, 2003). In the International Pediatric Adrenocortical Tumor Registry, which included adrenocortical adenomas in addition to carcinomas, diagnosis below age 4 years was associated with higher event-free survival (Michalkiewicz *et al.*, 2004). The excellent prognosis for carcinomas of the thyroid was typical of results in western populations (Shapiro and Bhattacharyya, 2005; Steliarova-Foucher *et al.*, 2006b). The lower survival for medullary compared with differentiated carcinoma was also found in ACCIS (Steliarova-Foucher *et al.*, 2006b). Nasopharyngeal carcinoma had a higher survival rate than in EUROCARE but that study only covered the first half of the 1990s (Gatta *et al.*, 2003). Skin carcinoma in children had a very high survival rate in ACCIS (de Vries *et al.*, 2006). Five-year survival of children with salivary gland carcinomas was already 71% in the 1970s (McWhirter *et al.*, 1989). The high survival rate for carcinoma of the lung is in striking contrast to the gloomy prognosis among adults; the majority of such tumours in children are low-grade bronchial adenomas (see Chapter 3). Carcinoma of the bladder in childhood is also often a low-grade tumour with excellent outcome, and it has been suggested that some of these tumours should for this reason not be classified as cancer (Fine *et al.*, 2005). In the only other published population-based series, children with carcinoid tumours of the appendix also had a very high survival rate (Parkes *et al.*, 1993).

The high survival rate for malignant melanoma was similar to that in the United States and Europe (Bernstein and Gurney, 1999; Conti *et al.*, 2001; de Vries *et al.*, 2006). In contrast to the present study, European survival rates for melanoma were similar in the two sexes (Conti *et al.*, 2001; de Vries *et al.*, 2006). The European studies also found high survival for ocular melanoma and low survival for melanoma of other noncutaneous sites (including the CNS) (Conti *et al.*, 2001; de Vries *et al.*, 2006).

5.2 Trends in survival

Figure 5.14 shows actuarial survival curves for children diagnosed with any type of cancer during successive quinquennia between 1966–1970 and 1996–2000. Five-year survival increased over the 30 years between these two periods from 28 to 76%. Survival increased by similarly large amounts for boys and girls (Table 5.15). There were large increases in survival in all age groups. Among children diagnosed during 1966–1970, survival was highest for infants and lowest for those aged 1–9 years at diagnosis. In every period since then, however, infants had a lower survival rate than older children. Consequently, the risk of death within 5 years from diagnosis was reduced by only 55% for infants, compared with 66–70% for older children.

Figures 5.15–5.26 show the actuarial survival curves for children diagnosed in each of the 12 groups of ICCC-3 during successive quinquennia. Five-year survival rates for children diagnosed in each of the 12 groups during 1966–1970 and 1996–2000 are shown in Table 5.16, together with the reduction in risk of death within 5 years from diagnosis between the two periods. Table 5.17 shows changes in risk of death among children diagnosed in successive quinquennia.

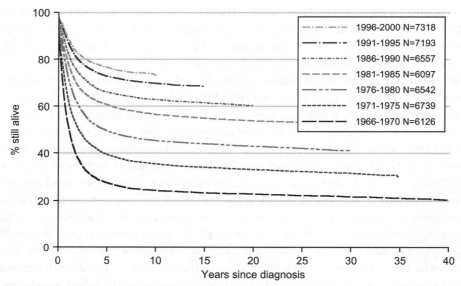

Fig. 5.14 Actuarial survival curves for children aged 0–14 years at diagnosis with all cancers combined, by five-year calendar period of diagnosis. Great Britain, 1966–2000.

Survival increased substantially for all diagnostic groups over the study period. The risk of dying within 5 years from diagnosis with any type of childhood cancer was reduced by two-thirds, and the reductions in risk for diagnostic groups ranged from around half for CNS tumours, neuroblastoma, etc., bone tumours and soft tissue sarcoma to more than three-quarters for leukaemias, lymphomas, renal tumours, germ cell and gonadal tumours and the miscellaneous group of other and unspecified malignant neoplasms (Table 5.16). The risk of death decreased by more than 10% between successive quinquennia of diagnosis for all cancers combined (Table 5.17). The risk also declined for most diagnostic groups between each pair of successive quinquennia.

Survival increased substantially between 1966–1970 and 1971–1975 for leukaemias, lymphomas, renal tumours and miscellaneous epithelial cancers, but for most diagnostic groups the major improvements in prognosis took place more recently. Apart from the rather small and heterogeneous groups of other epithelial neoplasms and melanoma, and other and unspecified malignant neoplasms, the only instance of a substantial increase in the risk of death between successive quinquennia of diagnosis affected children with renal tumours, for whom the risk increased by 38% between 1986–1990 and 1991–1995. This was followed, however, by a reduction in risk of 47% between 1991–1995 and 1996–2000. The net effect was a reduction of 27% in risk of death between 1986–1990 and 1996–2000.

Trends in survival during 1971 onwards for more detailed diagnostic categories are shown in Table 5.18. Survival increased significantly for almost all categories, the main exceptions being several types of CNS tumour. The increase in survival did not take place uniformly over the 30-year period, or at the same time for each type of cancer. For each

Text starts on page 180

Table 5.15 Trends in survival from childhood cancer diagnosed during 1966–2000. Five-year survival (%) by sex and age at diagnosis for children diagnosed in successive quinquennia, with change in risk of death between 1966–1970 and 1996–2000. N, total number of cases followed up. P, p-value from test for trend in survival by single calendar year of diagnosis

Category	N	1966–1970	1971–1975	1976–1980	1981–1985	1986–1990	1991–1995	1996–2000	P	Change in risk (%)
Total	46572	28	39	50	61	66	73	77	<0.0001	−67.5
Boys	25926	27	38	49	61	66	73	76	<0.0001	−67.0
Girls	20646	29	42	51	60	66	73	77	<0.0001	−68.1
Age 0	3971	35	37	46	54	60	67	71	<0.0001	−54.8
1–4	17256	25	40	49	62	67	74	77	<0.0001	−69.8
5–9	12634	26	40	50	62	66	74	77	<0.0001	−68.9
10–14	12711	31	38	50	60	67	71	77	<0.0001	−66.2

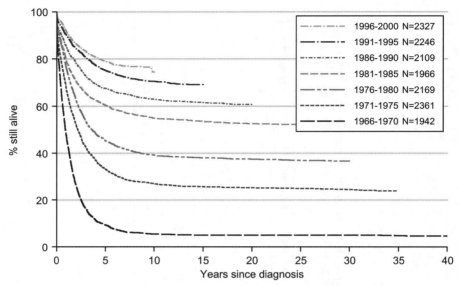

Fig. 5.15 Actuarial survival curves for children aged 0–14 years at diagnosis with leukaemia, by five-year calendar period of diagnosis. Great Britain, 1966–2000.

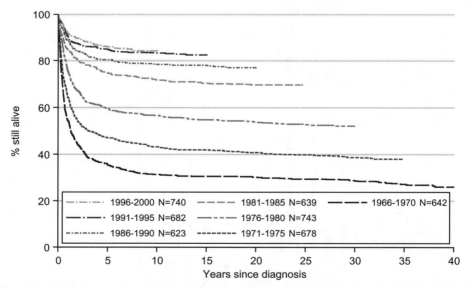

Fig. 5.16 Actuarial survival curves for children aged 0–14 years at diagnosis with lymphomas and reticuloendothelial neoplasms, by five-year calendar period of diagnosis. Great Britain, 1966–2000.

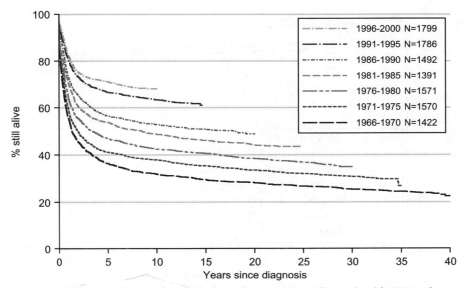

Fig. 5.17 Actuarial survival curves for children aged 0–14 years at diagnosis with CNS and miscellaneous intracranial and intraspinal neoplasms, by five-year calendar period of diagnosis. Great Britain, 1966–2000.

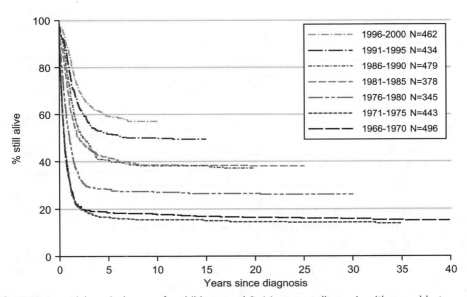

Fig. 5.18 Actuarial survival curves for children aged 0–14 years at diagnosis with neuroblastoma and other peripheral nervous cell tumours, by five-year calendar period of diagnosis. Great Britain, 1966–2000.

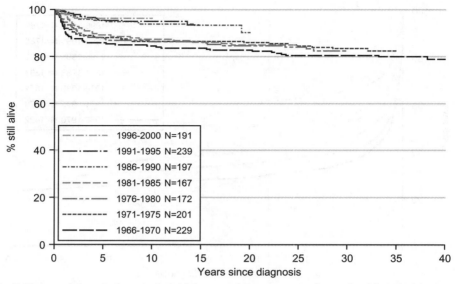

Fig. 5.19 Actuarial survival curves for children aged 0–14 years at diagnosis with retinoblastoma, by five-year calendar period of diagnosis. Great Britain, 1966–2000.

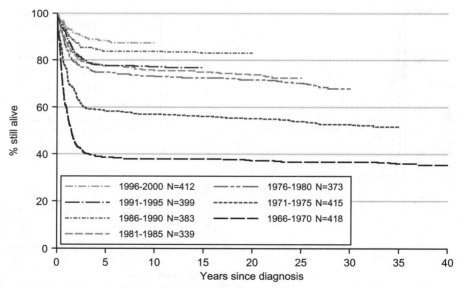

Fig. 5.20 Actuarial survival curves for children aged 0–14 years at diagnosis with renal tumours, by five-year calendar period of diagnosis. Great Britain, 1966–2000.

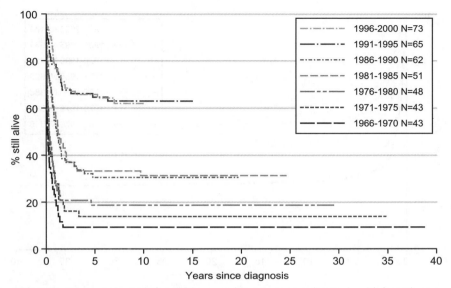

Fig. 5.21 Actuarial survival curves for children aged 0–14 years at diagnosis with hepatic tumours, by five-year calendar period of diagnosis. Great Britain, 1966–2000.

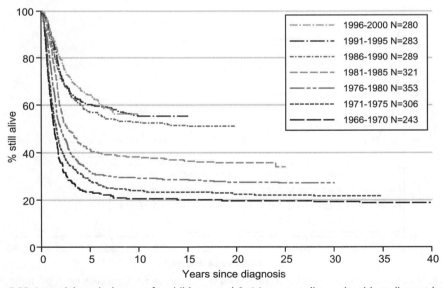

Fig. 5.22 Actuarial survival curves for children aged 0–14 years at diagnosis with malignant bone tumours, by five-year calendar period of diagnosis. Great Britain, 1966–2000.

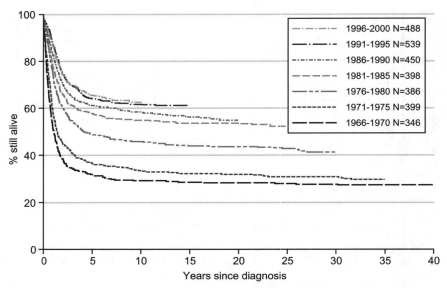

Fig. 5.23 Actuarial survival curves for children aged 0–14 years at diagnosis with soft tissue and other extraosseous sarcomas, by five-year calendar period of diagnosis. Great Britain, 1966–2000.

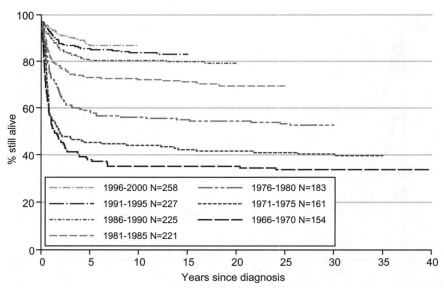

Fig. 5.24 Actuarial survival curves for children aged 0–14 years at diagnosis with germ cell tumours, trophoblastic tumours and neoplasms of gonads, by five-year calendar period of diagnosis. Great Britain, 1966–2000.

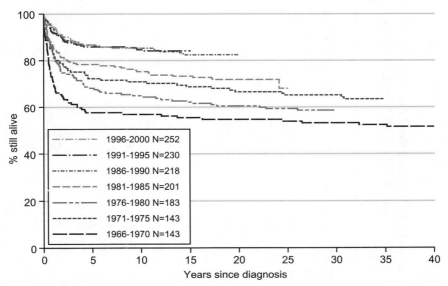

Fig. 5.25 Actuarial survival curves for children aged 0–14 years at diagnosis with other malignant epithelial neoplasms and malignant melanoma, by five-year calendar period of diagnosis. Great Britain, 1966–2000.

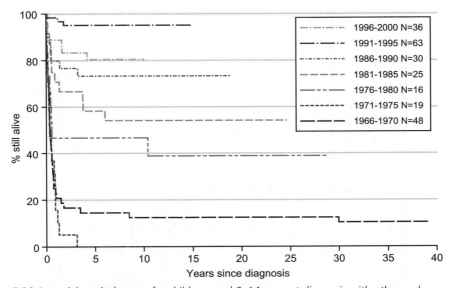

Fig. 5.26 Actuarial survival curves for children aged 0–14 years at diagnosis with other and unspecified malignant neoplasms, by five-year calendar period of diagnosis. Great Britain, 1966–2000.

Table 5.16 Trends in survival from childhood cancer diagnosed during 1966–2000. Five-year survival rate for all cancers and the 12 main diagnostic groups of ICCC-3 among children diagnosed during successive quinquennia, with change in risk of death between 1966–1970 and 1996–2000. N, total number of cases followed up. P, p-value from test for trend in survival by single calendar year of diagnosis

Tumour type	N	Five-year survival (%)								P	Change in risk (%)
		1966–70	1971–75	1976–80	1981–85	1986–90	1991–95	1996–2000			
All cancers	46572	28	39	50	61	66	73	77	<0.0001	−67.5
Leukaemias	15120	9	33	45	60	68	75	79	<0.0001	−76.9
Lymphomas	4747	36	47	59	75	81	85	86	<0.0001	−78.4
CNS tumours	11031	37	41	47	54	57	67	71	<0.0001	−54.5
Neuroblastoma, etc.	3037	19	17	28	42	41	52	59	<0.0001	−50.2
Retinoblastoma	1396	86	88	88	89	95	95	96	<0.0001	−73.8
Renal tumours	2739	39	59	75	78	84	78	88	<0.0001	−80.6
Hepatic tumours	385	9	14	19	33	31	65	66	<0.0001	−62.2
Bone tumours	2075	23	28	32	41	57	60	64	<0.0001	−53.3
Soft tissue sarcomas	3006	32	37	49	58	61	64	66	<0.0001	−49.4
Germ cell and gonadal	1429	38	45	59	73	80	85	87	<0.0001	−78.7
Other epithelial & melanoma	1370	58	72	68	78	87	86	87	<0.0001	−68.9
Other and unspecified	237	15	0	47	58	73	95	81	<0.0001	−77.2

Table 5.17 Change in risk of death within 5 years from diagnosis (%) for all cancers and the 12 main diagnostic groups of ICCC-3 among children diagnosed during successive quinquennia between 1966–1970 and 1996–2000

Periods of diagnosis	1966–70, 1971–75	1971–75, 1976–80	1976–80, 1981–85	1981–85, 1986–90	1986–90, 1991–95	1991–95, 1996–2000
All cancers	−16.2	−16.7	−22.1	−13.4	−19.7	−14.0
Leukaemias	−26.3	−18.2	−27.7	−17.9	−23.5	−15.7
Lymphomas	−17.9	−23.3	−37.8	−22.8	−22.8	−7.3
CNS tumours	−7.4	−9.9	−13.3	−5.8	−22.8	−13.6
Neuroblastoma, etc.	+2.3	−12.7	−19.6	+1.4	−18.4	−16.1
Retinoblastoma	−15.3	−1.3	−8.4	−57.5	+0.2	−19.8
Renal tumours	−32.4	−39.2	−11.0	−27.7	+37.6	−46.7
Hepatic tumours	−5.1	−5.6	−17.9	+4.0	−49.0	−3.2
Bone tumours	−6.4	−5.2	−13.8	−26.4	−7.7	−10.1
Soft tissue sarcomas	−6.9	−19.0	−17.6	−8.2	−7.6	−4.0
Germ cell and gonadal	−12.0	−24.9	−34.6	−27.0	−25.8	−9.1
Other epithelial and melanoma	−34.7	+15.0	−32.1	−38.5	+5.7	−6.3
Other	+17.1	−53.3	−21.9	−36.0	−81.7	+397.5

Table 5.18 Trends in survival from childhood cancer in Britain, 1971–2000. Numbers of cases followed up (N), five-year survival rates (%) for children diagnosed during successive calendar periods, and P-value from test for trend in survival by single calendar year of diagnosis over the period for which survival rates are shown

Diagnostic category	N	1971–75	1976–80	1981–85	1986–90	1991–95	1996–2000	1971–80	1981–90	1991–2000	P
Lymphoid leukaemias	10539	41	53	69	74	81	83				<0.0001
Precursor cell leukaemias	10421	41	53	70	75	81	83				<0.0001
CD10 Positive	5433	–	64	77	81	86	87				<0.0001
Null cell	384	–	46	52	51	59	58				0.0418
T-cell	923	–	32	42	51	62	71				<0.0001
Mature B-cell leukaemias	100	–	–	38	41	71	78				<0.0001
Acute myeloid leukaemias	2094	6	14	26	44	51	65				<0.0001
Chronic myeloid leukaemia	196	21	22	52	32	48	67				<0.0001
JMML/CMML	124	14	11	0	26	32	33				0.0021
Unspecified and other specified leukaemias	156	–	18	16	36	59	73				<0.0001
Hodgkin lymphomas	1715	80	86	90	91	96	94				<0.0001
Non-Hodgkin lymphomas (including Burkitt lymphoma)	2266	24	41	65	74	78	81				<0.0001
Ependymomas and choroid plexus tumour	1027	35	29	50	44	66	64				<0.0001
Ependymomas	846	36	30	51	40	64	69				<0.0001

	N							p
Astrocytomas	3825	56	63	69	71	76	81	<0.0001
Low grade	2577	75	78	82	84	91	93	<0.0001
High grade	567	13	15	25	20	18	16	0.1027
Intracranial and intraspinal embryonal tumours	1947	25	35	42	42	45	55	<0.0001
Medulloblastomas	1636	26	35	46	45	52	65	<0.0001
Primitive neuroectodermal tumour (PNET)	230	–	–	–	30	23	32	0.5043
Other gliomas	1297	25	28	29	34	41	43	<0.0001
Oligodendrogliomas	142				57	56	72	0.0616
Mixed and unspecified gliomas	1139	21	24	24	30	37	41	<0.0001
Tumours of the sellar region (craniopharyngiomas)	500	67	72	88	93	89	99	<0.0001
Pineal parenchymal tumours	128				37	45	55	0.1363
Meningiomas	131				74	81	90	0.0591
Unspecified intracranial and intraspinal neoplasms	393	–	34	39	52	72	69	<0.0001
Neuroblastoma and ganglioneuroblastoma	2499	16	28	42	40	52	59	<0.0001
Retinoblastoma	1167	88	88	89	95	95	96	<0.0001
Unilateral	728	89	87	91	95	97	96	0.0017
Bilateral	418	85	90	86	95	93	97	0.0017

Table 5.18 (continued) Trends in survival from childhood cancer in Britain, 1971–2000. Numbers of cases followed up (N), five-year survival rates (%) for children diagnosed during successive calendar periods, and P-value from test for trend in survival by single calendar year of diagnosis over the period for which survival rates are shown

Diagnostic category	N	1971–75	1976–80	1981–85	1986–90	1991–95	1996–2000	1971–80	1981–90	1991–2000	P
Nephroblastoma and other nonepithelial renal tumours	2269	59	76	78	84	78	88				<0.0001
Nephroblastoma	2151	59	76	80	84	80	91				<0.0001
Rhabdoid renal tumour	42							–	28	25	0.4131
Clear cell sarcoma of kidney	49							–	84	75	0.7720
Hepatoblastoma	265	14	21	41	37	70	79				<0.0001
Hepatic carcinomas	75							11	16	20	0.5876
Osteosarcomas	979	21	30	42	50	53	62				<0.0001
Ewing tumour and related bone sarcomas	624	–	33	41	63	66	63				<0.0001
Rhabdomyosarcomas	1583	31	44	58	58	64	68				<0.0001
Fibrosarcomas, peripheral nerve sheath tumours and other fibrous neoplasms	247	58	43	63	75	73	68				0.0008
Fibroblastic and myofibroblastic tumours	161							60	73	83	0.0009
Fibrohistiocytic tumours	83							–	83	96	0.0398
Unspecified soft	189	31	59	27	53	48	42				0.0906

tissue sarcomas

Diagnostic group	N							p-value
Intracranial and intraspinal germ cell tumours	364	48	49	65	55	77	81	<0.0001
Malignant extracranial and extragonadal germ cell tumours	164	–	–		82	80	79	0.7826
Malignant gonadal germ cell tumours	595	52	70	86	94	97	96	<0.0001
Testicular	298	60	71	88	97	100	98	<0.0001
Ovarian	297	43	69	85	90	93	94	<0.0001
Adrenocortical carcinomas	70				25	39	50	0.0082
Thyroid carcinomas	182	100	96	100	93	100	100	0.1506
Nasopharyngeal carcinomas	99				57	42	83	0.0361
Malignant melanomas	305	–	72	85	93	91	85	0.0105
Skin carcinomas	213	100	96	100	100	97	100	0.5115
Other and unspecified carcinomas	336	60	55	74	79	74	79	0.0023
Carcinomas of salivary glands	53				96	97	–	0.2598
Carcinomas of other specified sites	81				88	79	–	0.6243

diagnostic category in Table 5.18 for which the trend in survival over time was signifi-cant, the successive quinquennia between which five-year survival increased by the great-est number of percentage points are shown in Table 5.19, and the successive quinquennia with the greatest proportional reduction in the risk of death within 5 years are shown in Table 5.20.

By both measures, the greatest improvement in prognosis overall took place between 1976–1980 and 1981–1985. This was also the period that saw the biggest advances in sur-vival and reductions in mortality for children with leukaemia, particularly precursor-cell ALL and CML, and also for those with NHL and rhabdomyosarcoma. For AML, the largest increment in survival was between 1981–1985 and 1986–1990, while the greatest reduction in risk of death was between 1991–1995 and 1996–2000. For Hodgkin lym-phomas and renal tumours, the largest increases in five-year survival took place between the earlier and later 1970s, but the risk of death fell most markedly in the 1990s. As noted above, however, the improved survival for renal tumours in the later 1990s was preceded by a worsening of prognosis in the first half of the decade.

The largest increment in survival for neuroblastoma, 13.7 percentage points, occurred between 1976–1980 and 1981–1985, but there was also a substantial increase of 11.5 per-centage points between 1986–1990 and 1991–1995. The decreases in the risk of death in these two periods were very similar, 19.1 and 19.2%, respectively.

For other diagnostic groups and subgroups, the main improvements in prognosis occurred relatively recently, with especially large increases in survival and/or decrease in risk of death for retinoblastoma, Ewing tumour of bone and gonadal germ cell tumours in the later 1980s, AML in the later 1980s and earlier 1990s, and hepatoblastoma also in the earlier 1990s. Advances in survival for children with CNS tumours were mostly less spectacular and tended also to be relatively recent.

The period covered by this study saw important changes in the organization of the care and treatment of children with cancer. By the early 1970s, there were a few specialist regional treatment centres with a paediatric oncology team (UKCCSG, 2002). This model spread throughout the British Isles with the formation of the UKCCSG in 1977 and its subsequent expansion (Mott et al., 1997; Barnes, 2005). By the late 1990s, more than 85% of children with cancer were referred to a paediatric oncology centre affiliated to the UKCCSG (UKCCSG, 2002).

In the early 1970s, substantial numbers of children with ALL and renal tumours were entered in national clinical trials under the auspices of the Medical Research Council (Medical Research Council's Working Party on Leukaemia in Childhood, 1977; Medical Research Council's Working Party on Embryonal Tumours in Childhood, 1978; Lennox et al., 1979; Stiller and Draper, 1989). A few children with Hodgkin lymphoma were included in the British National Lymphoma Investigation (Makepeace et al., 1987). The Medical Research Council sponsored trials for AML in parallel with those for ALL, but few children were entered until the start of the first trial specifically for childhood AML opened at the end of 1974 (Chessells et al., 1983; Stiller and Eatock, 1994). Several centres entered children in the first SIOP medulloblastoma trial (Tait et al., 1990) and the first MRC osteosarcoma trial (Medical Research Council working party on bone sarcoma, 1986), both

Text starts on page 187

Table 5.19 Successive quinquennia of diagnosis during 1971–2000 between which the increase in five-year survival was greatest, with size of increase

Diagnostic category	Years of diagnosis	Increase in survival (percentage points)
All cancers	1976–80, 1981–85	11.1
Leukaemias, myeloproliferative and myelodysplastic diseases		
Lymphoid leukaemias	1976–80, 1981–85	15.1
Precursor cell leukaemias	1976–80, 1981–85	16.3
CD10 Positive	1976–80, 1981–85	16.8
Null cell	1976–80, 1981–85	15.5
T-cell	1986–90, 1991–95	8.4
Mature B-cell leukaemias	1986–90, 1991–95	10.6
Acute myeloid leukaemias	1986–90, 1991–95	30.1
Chronic myeloid leukaemia	1981–85, 1986–90	18.1
JMML/CMML	1976–80, 1981–85	29.8
Unspecified and other specified leukaemias	1981–85, 1986–90	26.3
	1986–90, 1991–95	23.5
Lymphomas and reticuloendothelial neoplasms	1976–80, 1981–85	15.3
Hodgkin lymphomas	1971–75, 1976–80	6.7
Non-Hodgkin lymphomas (including Burkitt lymphoma)	1976–80, 1981–85	23.8
CNS and miscellaneous intracranial and intraspinal neoplasms	1986–90, 1991–95	9.9
Ependymomas	1986–90, 1991–95	23.9
Astrocytomas	1971–75, 1976–80	6.9
Low grade	1986–90, 1991–95	7.0
Medulloblastomas	1991–95, 1996–2000	12.2
Mixed and unspecified gliomas	1986–90, 1991–95	6.7
Tumours of the sellar region (craniopharyngiomas)	1976–80, 1981–85	15.7

Table 5.19 (continued) Successive quinquennia of diagnosis during 1971–2000 between which the increase in five-year survival was greatest, with size of increase

Diagnostic category	Years of diagnosis	Increase in survival (percentage points)
Unspecified intracranial and intraspinal neoplasms	1986–90, 1991–95	21.7
Neuroblastoma and other peripheral nervous cell tumours		
Neuroblastoma and ganglioneuroblastoma	1976–80, 1981–85	13.2
	1976–80, 1981–85	13.7
Retinoblastoma		
Unilateral	1981–85, 1986–90	6.2
	1981–85, 1986–90	4.6
Bilateral	1981–85, 1986–90	8.8
Renal tumours	1971–75, 1976–80	16.3
Nephroblastoma and other nonepithelial renal tumours	1971–75, 1976–80	16.8
Nephroblastoma	1971–75, 1976–80	16.9
Hepatic tumours	1986–90, 1991–95	34.0
Hepatoblastoma	1986–90, 1991–95	33.2
Malignant bone tumours	1981–85, 1986–90	15.5
Osteosarcomas	1976–80, 1981–85	12.0
Ewing tumour and related bone sarcomas	1981–85, 1986–90	22.1

Soft tissue and other extraosseous sarcomas	1971–75, 1976–80	12.0
Rhabdomyosarcomas	1976–80, 1981–85	13.7
Fibrosarcomas, peripheral nerve sheath tumours and other fibrous neoplasms	1976–80, 1981–85	19.3
Germ cell tumours, trophoblastic tumours and neoplasms of gonads	1976–80, 1981–85	14.2
Intracranial and intraspinal germ cell tumours	1986–90, 1991–95	21.3
Malignant gonadal germ cell tumours	1971–75, 1976–80	18.7
Testicular	1976–80, 1981–85	16.1
Ovarian	1971–75, 1976–80	26.2
Other malignant epithelial neoplasms and malignant melanomas	1976–80, 1981–85	10.2
Malignant melanomas	1976–80, 1981–85	12.2
Other and unspecified carcinomas	1976–80, 1981–85	19.4
Other and unspecified malignant neoplasms	1986–90, 1991–95	21.8

Table 5.20 Successive quinquennia of diagnosis during 1971–2000, between which the percentage reduction in risk of death within 5 years from diagnosis was greatest, along with the size of reduction

Diagnostic category	Years of diagnosis	Change in risk (%)
All cancers	1976–80, 1981–85	–22.1
Leukaemias, myeloproliferative and myelodysplastic diseases	1976–80, 1981–85	–27.7
Lymphoid leukaemias	1976–80, 1981–85	–34.6
Precursor cell leukaemias	1976–80, 1981–85	–35.3
CD10 Positive	1976–80, 1981–85	–39.9
Null cell	1986–90, 1991–95	–17.0
T-cell	1991–95, 1996–2000	–23.0
Mature B-cell leukaemias	1986–90, 1991–95	–50.9
Acute myeloid leukaemias	1991–95, 1996–2000	–29.1
Chronic myeloid leukaemia	1976–80, 1981–85	–38.3
JMML/CMML	1981–85, 1986–90	–26.3
Unspecified and other specified leukaemias	1986–90, 1991–95	–36.6
Lymphomas and reticuloendothelial neoplasms	1976–80, 1981–85	–37.8
Hodgkin lymphomas	1986–90, 1991–95	–55.9
Non-Hodgkin lymphomas (including Burkitt lymphoma)	1976–80, 1981–85	–40.2
CNS and miscellaneous intracranial and intraspinal neoplasms	1986–90, 1991–95	–22.8
Ependymomas	1986–90, 1991–95	–39.9

Astrocytomas	1986–90, 1991–95	−19.7
Low grade	1986–90, 1991–95	−43.7
Medulloblastomas	1991–95, 1996–2000	−25.6
Mixed and unspecified gliomas	1986–90, 1991–95	−9.6
Tumours of the sellar region (craniopharyngiomas)	1991–95, 1996–2000	−90.3
Unspecified intracranial and intraspinal neoplasms	1986–90, 1991–95	−41.8
Neuroblastoma and other peripheral nervous cell tumours	1976–80, 1981–85	−18.5
Neuroblastoma and ganglioneuroblastoma	1976–80, 1981–85	−19.2
Retinoblastoma	1981–85, 1986–90	−57.5
Unilateral	1981–85, 1986–90	−50.2
Bilateral	1981–85, 1986–90	−65.1
Renal tumours	1991–95, 1996–2000	−46.7
Nephroblastoma and other nonepithelial renal tumours	1991–95, 1996–2000	−45.9
Nephroblastoma	1991–95, 1996–2000	−57.1
Hepatic tumours	1986–90, 1991–95	−49.0
Hepatoblastoma	1986–90, 1991–95	−52.8
Malignant bone tumours	1981–85, 1986–90	−26.4
Osteosarcomas	1991–95, 1996–2000	−20.2
Ewing tumour and related bone sarcomas	1981–85, 1986–90	−37.5
Soft tissue and other extraosseous sarcomas	1971–75, 1976–80	−19.0
Rhabdomyosarcomas	1976–80, 1981–85	−24.5
Fibrosarcomas, peripheral nerve sheath tumours and other fibrous neoplasms	1976–80, 1981–85	−33.9

Table 5.20 (continued) Successive quinquennia of diagnosis during 1971–2000, between which the percentage reduction in risk of death within 5 years from diagnosis was greatest, along with the size of reduction

Diagnostic category	Years of diagnosis	Change in risk (%)
Germ cell tumours, trophoblastic tumours and neoplasms of gonads		
Intracranial and intraspinal germ cell tumours	1976–80, 1981–85	–34.6
	1986–90, 1991–95	–47.5
Malignant gonadal germ cell tumours	1981–85, 1986–90	–55.9
Testicular	1981–85, 1986–90*	–72.4
Ovarian	1976–80, 1981–85	–49.8
Other malignant epithelial neoplasms and malignant melanomas	1981–85, 1986–90	–38.5
Malignant melanomas	1981–85, 1986–90	–57.6
Other and unspecified carcinomas	1976–80, 1981–85	–42.8
Other and unspecified malignant neoplasms	1986–90, 1991–95	–81.7

* Risk of death fell by 100% between 1986–90 and 1991–95, but this was based on only two deaths for the earlier period.

of which began in 1975. Clinical trial activity in paediatric oncology in the UK increased greatly with the development of the UKCCSG. The group's first trials, for NHL and T-cell ALL, began in 1977 (Mott *et al.*, 1984a,b). By the 1990s, it was organizing national protocols or participating in international trials for nearly all the principal childhood malignancies other than leukaemia (Ablett *et al.*, 2003).

The most important improvements in survival for many childhood cancers in Britain coincided with the eras of key clinical trials and show the impact of these trials on population-based survival. For ALL, the notable increase in survival in 1981–1985 over the previous quinquennium occurred in parallel with the improved results from the UKALL VIII trial, which was open from 1980 to 1984 (The Medical Research Council, 1986; Stiller and Draper, 1989; Eden *et al.*, 1991). There was a considerable further increase in survival between 1986–1990 and 1991–1995. This corresponded approximately to the transition from UKALL X (1985–1990) to UKALL XI (1990–1997), with eight-year survival increasing between the two trials from 74 to 81% (Chessells *et al.*, 2002c). Event-free survival, however, was identical in the two trials (Chessells *et al.*, 2002c), indicating the major contribution of more effective treatment for relapsed ALL in the UKALL R1 study (Lawson *et al.*, 2000; Chessells *et al.*, 2002c). Survival of infants with ALL who were included in the trials for children of all ages before 1990 was very poor (Chessells *et al.*, 1994). Their outlook improved with the development of specific treatment protocols for infants, but they remain a poor prognosis group (Chessells *et al.*, 2002b).

Mature B-cell leukaemia has been treated in a similar way to B-cell NHL for the past two decades (Hann *et al.*, 1990); the very large increase in survival in the 1990s reflects the success of the 1990 protocol in this disease (Atra *et al.*, 1998).

The outlook for children with AML has improved dramatically, with five-year survival increasing from 6% for those diagnosed during 1971–1975 to 65% by 1996–2000. Large increases in survival have also taken place within the national AML trials, especially since the mid-1980s (Gibson *et al.*, 2005). When the main results were published from AML10, which was open from 1988 to 1995, they were better than those of any previous childhood AML trial worldwide (Stevens *et al.*, 1998). Treatment-related mortality fell by nearly half during the course of AML10 (Riley *et al.*, 1999). Overall survival increased further in AML12 compared to AML10 (Gibson *et al.*, 2005).

Survival rates for children with Hodgkin lymphoma were already high in the early 1970s. Therefore, the subsequent increase in survival, though statistically significant, has necessarily been relatively small. The more impressive reductions in risk of death, especially by more than 50% in the early 1990s, have presumably resulted from improved survival for poor-prognosis subgroups, especially children with stage IV disease. The first two UKCCSG Hodgkin's disease studies were open during 1982–1992 and 1992–1999, respectively, but stage IV patients received the same treatment in both studies (Atra *et al.*, 2002). Results have not been published for the more recent study separately, but the ten-year survival rates of 71% in the first study (Shankar *et al.*, 1997) and 77% in the two studies combined (Atra *et al.*, 2002) suggest that outcome was considerably better in the second study.

The UKCCSG ran three successive series of NHL studies starting in 1977 (Mott *et al.*, 1984a,b), 1985 (Hann *et al.*, 1990; Pinkerton *et al.*, 1991; Eden *et al.*, 1992; Burke *et al.*, 2003) and 1990 (Atra *et al.*, 1998, 2000; Burke *et al.*, 2003). Although there was a pronounced increase in population-based survival during the period of the first series of studies, this continued during the period of the second series, which finished in 1990. These increases reflect further progress within the studies themselves; for example, four-year event-free survival for T-cell NHL increased from 40% in the first series (Mott *et al.*, 1984a) to 65% in the second (Eden *et al.*, 1992). Increases in population-based survival for childhood NHL since 1990, although less dramatic, were consistent with the improvements achieved in the 1990 series of studies (Atra *et al.*, 1998, 2000).

Survival increased steadily for medulloblastoma throughout the 30-year study period, except for a pause during the 1980s. The resumption of the trend in the 1990s reflects the improved outcome in the SIOP/UKCCSG PNET-3 study (Taylor *et al.*, 2003) compared with SIOP II (Bailey *et al.*, 1995). There is no obvious explanation, however, for the especially large increase in survival between the earlier and later 1990s, since PNET-3 was open during most of that decade and no change in outcome during the course of the trial has been reported (Taylor *et al.*, 2003). Within PNET-3, as in contemporary population-based data, results for other PNET were inferior to those for medulloblastoma (Pizer *et al.*, 2006).

In the absence of any sizeable increase in incidence of good-prognosis neuroblastoma, for example by increased frequency of incidental diagnosis, increases in the overall survival rate for neuroblastoma must largely reflect improved outcome for poor-prognosis cases, preeminently metastatic disease in children aged 1 year and above. Stage 4 neuroblastoma was for many years one of the most intractable diseases in paediatric oncology. The first substantial improvement in neuroblastoma prognosis occurred in the early 1980s, around the time of the first ENSG clinical trial (Pritchard *et al.*, 2005). There was then no further progress in survival until the 1990s, when five-year survival for all neuroblastoma combined at last exceeded 50%. Large numbers of children over the age of 1 year with stage 4 disease were entered in the ENSG-5 trial (Pearson *et al.*, 1994); their results have not yet been reported.

Five-year survival from retinoblastoma already exceeded 85% in the mid-1960s. The only appreciable increase since then occurred in the second half of the 1980s, when five-year survival reached 95% and the risk of death within 5 years of diagnosis was reduced by more than half compared with the previous quinquennium. Retinoblastoma, unusually, had not been the subject of any national or multicentre trials up to that time. Treatment was already highly centralized, however, with 40% of children diagnosed during 1969–80 being referred to a single centre in London (Sanders *et al.*, 1988). The marked increase in survival in the later 1980s was probably related to the development of more effective treatment for the small minority of poor-prognosis patients (Kingston *et al.*, 1996; Madreperla *et al.*, 1998).

Survival of children with renal tumours, and nephroblastoma in particular, increased steadily until about 1980, presumably as a result of increasingly effective chemotherapy both within and outside the MRC trials (Medical Research Council's Working Party on Embryonal Tumours in Childhood, 1978; Lennox *et al.*, 1979; Pritchard *et al.*, 1995). Thereafter, the pattern was more complicated, with an increase in survival in the second half of the 1980s, followed in the earlier 1990s by reversion to the survival rate of 10 years before, and then in turn by an increase in survival in the later 1990s to the highest levels yet achieved. The pattern in the 1980s is inconsistent with that of the first two UKCCSG Wilms' tumour studies, which were open to entry during 1980–1986 and 1986–1991, respectively. Survival was similar in the two trials for children with unilateral, non-metastatic tumours of favourable histology and for those with anaplastic histology in all stages combined, while the second trial showed a distinct improvement over the first in outcome for stage IV patients with favourable histology (Pritchard *et al.*, 1995; Mitchell *et al.*, 2000). The third UKCCSG study was in progress throughout the 1990s, and there was a large reduction in the risk of death between the first and second halves of the decade in the population-based data. Unless there were marked differences in histology or stage distribution between the two periods, it seems most likely that the improved prognosis reflected more effective treatment for relapsed Wilms' tumour. Clear cell sarcoma of the kidney, formerly known as bone metastasizing renal tumour of childhood, was traditionally classified as an unfavourable histology for renal tumours; the high survival achieved by the beginning of the 1980s confirmed in population data the findings of clinical trials that modern chemotherapy is highly effective against this tumour (Pritchard *et al.*, 1995). In contrast, the very low population survival for rhabdoid renal tumour corroborates the still dismal results of recent clinical studies (Mitchell *et al.*, 2000).

For many years, hepatoblastoma had an extremely poor prognosis, with survival even lower than for neuroblastoma. This changed dramatically in the early 1990s, when five-year survival suddenly increased to over 70%. The very large improvement in prognosis was undoubtedly linked to the success of the first SIOP hepatoblastoma study, in which a large proportion of British patients were entered (Pritchard *et al.*, 2000).

While survival increased for sarcomas of bone and soft tissue, the improvements were moderate compared with some other paediatric cancers. For osteosarcoma, survival increased until the mid-1980s concurrently with the development and diffusion of relatively effective combination chemotherapy (Medical Research Council working party on bone sarcoma, 1986; Gill *et al.*, 1988; Bramwell *et al.*, 1992). The lack of progress during the next 10 years, when treatment remained essentially unchanged, has been documented not only among children but over the entire age range below 40 years (Stiller *et al.*, 2006c). In the most recent quinquennium of the study period, although there was no change in the proportion of children dying within 1 year from diagnosis, the three-year and five-year survival rates both increased by 9 percentage points, suggesting that further progress has been made in treating patients of intermediate prognosis. The largest increase in survival for Ewing sarcoma also occurred in the mid-1980s and patients of all ages below 40 years benefited from the improved survival (Stiller *et al.*, 2006c). The timing of the increase suggests that it was associated with the second national trial for Ewing sarcoma (Craft *et al.*, 1998).

The greatest increase in survival for rhabdomyosarcoma occurred between 1976–1980 and 1981–1985, a period that saw notable advances in the efficacy of multimodality therapy for this tumour (Maurer *et al.*, 1993). After a pause in the later 1980s, survival then increased steadily during the 1990s, though at a slower rate, in line with the more modest progress made in recent trials (Carli *et al.*, 2004; Stevens *et al.*, 2005).

The greatest increase in population-based survival for gonadal germ cell tumours took place during the 1970s, when the use of chemotherapy became widespread. The regimens used at that time were soon recognized to be inadequate, however, and the greatest proportional reduction in risk of death was in 1986–1990 compared to 1981–1985, around the time that the UKCCSG study adopted the BEP regimen that combined greater antitumour activity with an acceptably low frequency of fatal complications (Mann et al., 1989). By this time, five-year survival was well over 90%, leaving little room for further improvement.

The three largest population-based studies covering trends in survival from childhood cancer in other countries are those of EUROCARE (Gatta et al., 2005) and ACCIS (Steliarova-Foucher et al., 2004; Magnani et al., 2006) in Europe and the SEER Program (Jemal et al., 2005) in the United States. The calendar periods and presentation of results differ between the three studies. Nevertheless, some common patterns are easily seen, particularly the impressive gains in survival for gonadal germ cell tumours, ALL and NHL, and the relative lack of progress for soft tissue sarcomas and CNS tumours. Among childhood cancers that have not already been discussed because they have not been the subject of clinical trials in Britain, adrenocortical carcinoma and nasopharyngeal carcinoma showed impressive gains in the EUROCARE study as well as in Britain (Gatta et al., 2005). Children with chondrosarcoma also had a larger reduction in the risk of death in the EUROCARE study (Gatta et al., 2005), but there were too few British cases for analysis.

5.3 Long-term survival

So far, the presentation and discussion of trends in survival has concentrated on the first 5 years after diagnosis. This is when most deaths related to childhood cancer take place, and when the largest numbers of deaths have been prevented by advances in treatment. There is, however, still an important risk of death beyond 5 years from diagnosis, largely attributable to the original childhood cancer, subsequent malignancy or treatment-related causes (Robertson et al., 1994; Mertens et al., 2001; Möller et al., 2001). Table 5.21 shows trends in subsequent survival among children who had already survived 5 years. For all cancers combined, there was a continuing reduction in the risk of later death among five-year survivors. This pattern was also observed for leukaemias and lymphomas. For CNS tumours, the risk of death within 30 years of diagnosis among five-year survivors diagnosed during 1971–75 was 18% less than for those diagnosed during 1966–70. There was then no further reduction of mortality among five-year survivors until the later 1980s. For neuroblastoma, the improving trend in longer term survival of five-year survivors was interrupted by a large rise in the risk of later death for children diagnosed during 1981–85. As noted above, however, this was a period when there was a larger increase in five-year survival, and it seems likely that some deaths that would previously have occurred within 5 years were now being postponed. The overall effect was an increase in the probability of surviving 20 years from diagnosis, from 26% for 1976–80 to 38% for 1981–85. The fluctuating patterns of changing risk for children diagnosed in earlier years meant that there was no real improvement in the chances of

Table 5.21 Trends in subsequent survival among five-year survivors of childhood cancer. Survival probability (%) conditional on five-year survival by quinquennium of diagnosis, and percentage change in risk of death compared to the previous quinquennium

Calendar period of diagnosis		1966–70	1971–75	1971–75	1976–80	1976–80	1981–85	1981–85	1986–90	1986–90	1991–95
Total follow-up (years)		30	30	25	25	20	20	15	15	10	10
All cancers	Survival	79	80	82	85	87	89	91	93	95	96
	Change in risk		−6.4		−16.1		−15.8		−27.6		−14.1
Leukaemias	Survival	54	74	75	81	83	87	89	91	93	94
	Change in risk		−43.6		−24.7		−26.1		−23.4		−9.9
Lymphomas	Survival	81	82	85	89	91	93	94	97	97	98
	Change in risk		−6.9		−26.8		−26.5		−48.9		−27.2
CNS tumours	Survival	70	75	78	78	82	82	86	90	93	95
	Change in risk		−17.5		−1.9		−0.5		−30.2		−27.9
Neuroblastoma, etc.	Survival	86	87	87	93	94	92	92	94	94	96
	Change in risk		−6.0		−44.6		+32.0		−20.5		−42.2
Retinoblastoma	Survival	94	95	96	95	96	95	97	98	98	100
	Change in risk		−17.3		+17.5		+16.6		−36.0		−72.9
Renal tumours	Survival	95	90	92	94	96	95	97	99	100	99
	Change in risk		+95.3		−21.6		+15.8		−72.4		*
Hepatic tumours	Survival	100	100	100	100	100	94	94	100	100	98
	Change in risk		*		*		*		−100.0		*

Table 5.21 (continued) Trends in subsequent survival among five-year survivors of childhood cancer. Survival probability (%) conditional on five-year survival by quinquennium of diagnosis, and percentage change in risk of death compared to the previous quinquennium

Calendar period of diagnosis		1966–70	1971–75	1971–75	1976–80	1976–80	1981–85	1981–85	1986–90	1986–90	1991–95
Total follow-up (years)		30	30	25	25	20	20	15	15	10	10
Bone tumours	Survival	82	77	78	85	86	86	88	90	93	92
	Change in risk		+32.1		−31.9		−3.8		−14.4		+13.1
Soft tissue sarcomas	Survival	87	85	85	88	90	92	93	92	95	96
	Change in risk		+17.5		−22.2		−27.7		+15.0		−20.9
Germ cell and gonadal	Survival	89	89	90	91	92	95	98	99	100	98
	Change in risk		+0.6		−1.4		−33.9		−77.5		*
Other epithelial and melanoma	Survival	92	90	90	87	89	92	94	95	98	98
	Change in risk		+29.0		+30.2		−25.8		−23.3		−6.2
Other and unspecified	Survival	71	–	–	83	83	93	93	100	100	100
	Change in risk		–		–		−57.1		−100.0		*

*Change in risk could not be calculated because there were no deaths among five-year survivors diagnosed in the earlier period.– Survival could not be calculated because there were no five-year survivors.

continuing survival among five-year survivors of retinoblastoma or renal tumours diag-nosed before the later 1980s, or of germ cell and gonadal tumours diagnosed before the earlier 1980s. The late death rate for five-year survivors of hepatic tumours was very low throughout. Bone tumours and soft-tissue sarcomas also exhibited a fluctuating pattern of changing risk. There was little overall change for bone tumours, but the longer-term outlook for children with soft tissue sarcomas diagnosed in the earlier 1990s was some-what better than earlier.

These results show that, overall, the improvement in longer-term survival among five-year survivors of childhood cancer reported previously in Britain (Robertson *et al.*, 1994) has been sustained both with longer follow-up and into more recent periods of diagnosis. A sizeable decrease in late mortality of five-year survivors has also taken place in the Nordic countries, with a 39% reduction in the risk of later death among survivors diag-nosed in 1980–89 compared with 1960–79 (Möller *et al.*, 2001).

The increases in survival rates for almost all childhood cancers have led to correspon-ding increases in the number of long-term survivors in the population, and especially of adult survivors. The numbers of survivors in the British population have been estimated from the NRCT and, for persons diagnosed before 1962, from the series of survivors assembled from selected registries and treatment centres for long-term follow-up studies (Hawkins, 1989). A zero net effect of international migration has been assumed. The numbers should be regarded as minimum estimates because no adjustment has been made for possible underascertainment. The degree of underestimation is greater, how-ever, for survivors diagnosed before 1961, since the series from which they are derived, although ascertained in such a way as to minimize bias, makes no pretence of complete-ness. Figure 5.27 shows the estimated number of five-year survivors alive at the end of each year from 1971 to 2005. The total number increased over the 34-year period by a factor of 9.4, from 2753 to 25,989. The scale of the increase was more marked among older age groups. Table 5.22 shows the numbers of survivors at the end of 2005 by age group. Of the 25,989 five-year survivors known to be alive at the end of 2005, 17,167 were at least 20 years of age and 203 were aged 60 years and above. Figure 5.28–5.31 show the increase in numbers of five-year survivors for each of the 12 main diagnostic groups of ICCC-3. The largest increase was in five-year survivors of leukaemia, whose numbers were multiplied more than 100-fold. Table 5.22 also shows the numbers of five-year survivors at the end of 2005 by diagnostic group. Overall and in each age group below 40 years, survivors of leukaemia were most numerous. In each of the age groups from 40–69 years, survivors of brain and spinal tumours formed the largest diag-nostic group.

With the increase in the number and age of survivors of childhood cancer, recognition has grown of the wide range of medical and other problems that can affect them. The health and other aspects of these survivors are the subject of two very large and com-prehensive studies. In the United States, the multi-institutional Childhood Cancer Survivor Study (CCSS) has included over 20,000 survivors who were under 21 years of age when diagnosed with cancer up to 1986 (Robison *et al.*, 2002). The findings of the first 20 reports from the study have recently been summarized (Robison *et al.*, 2005).

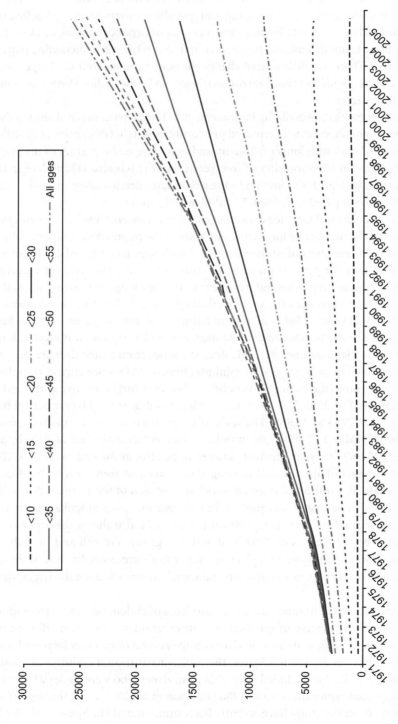

Fig. 5.27 Estimated numbers of five-year survivors of all childhood cancers combined alive at the end of successive calendar years, by attained age in years. Great Britain, 1971–2005.

Table 5.22 Estimated numbers of five-year survivors of childhood cancer in Great Britain who were alive at the end of 2005, by diagnostic group and attained age

Type of cancer	Age at end of 2005 (years)														
	5–9	10–14	15–19	20–24	25–29	30–34	35–39	40–44	45–49	50–54	55–59	60–64	65–69	70+	Total
Leukaemia	429	1297	1494	1362	1040	861	592	204	54	11	4	2	0	0	7350
Lymphoma	26	199	433	551	448	446	414	242	178	99	90	27	9	1	3163
CNS	190	616	967	928	621	576	570	446	296	243	148	49	10	2	5662
Neuroblastoma, etc.	183	216	199	159	106	65	77	84	46	24	9	3	1	0	1172
Retinoblastoma	126	200	201	155	144	158	182	147	102	76	46	13	5	6	1561
Renal tumours	143	290	342	269	250	256	206	136	85	47	20	4	4	0	2052
Hepatic tumours	30	39	23	22	11	10	5	3	1	0	1	0	0	0	145
Bone tumours	3	27	105	151	156	117	103	78	49	52	41	14	3	2	901
Soft tissue sarcomas	63	192	268	289	194	195	144	113	84	68	50	20	2	1	1683
Germ cell and gonadal	64	87	176	190	140	113	104	70	43	30	17	9	0	0	1042
Melanoma and carcinoma	16	38	113	214	152	175	111	102	78	63	32	10	2	0	1106
Other and unspecified	10	21	37	21	24	12	10	4	2	4	3	2	1	1	152
Total	**1283**	**3222**	**4358**	**4311**	**3286**	**2984**	**2517**	**1629**	**1018**	**717**	**461**	**153**	**37**	**13**	**25,989**

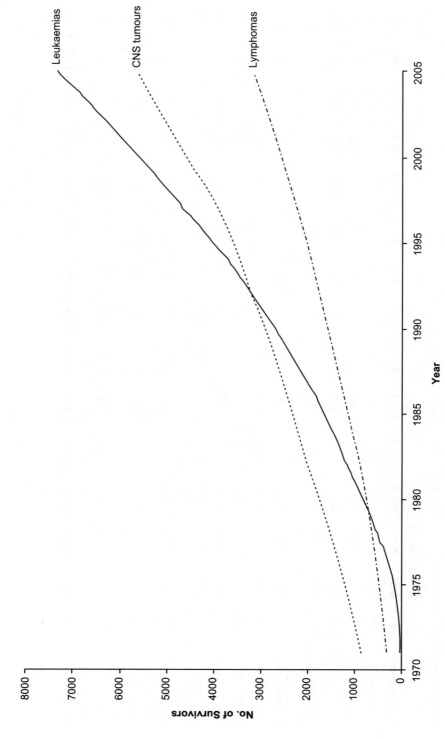

Fig. 5.28 Estimated numbers of five-year survivors of childhood leukaemias, lymphomas and CNS tumours alive at the end of successive calendar years, by diagnostic group. Great Britain, 1971–2005.

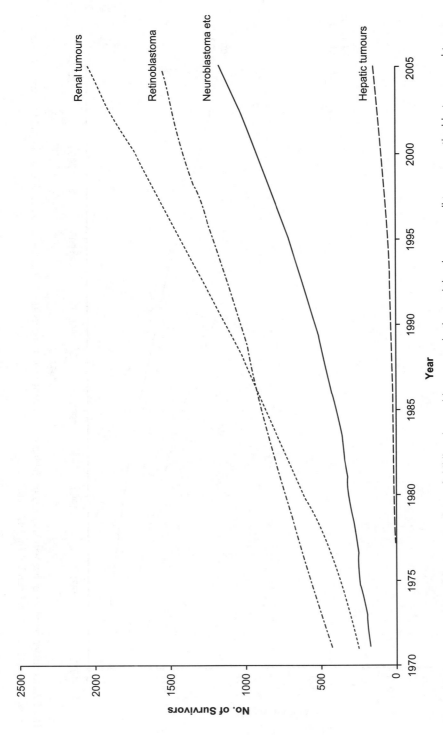

Fig. 5.29 Estimated numbers of five-year survivors of childhood neuroblastoma and other peripheral nervous cell tumours, retinoblastoma, renal tumours and hepatic tumours alive at the end of successive calendar years, by diagnostic group. Great Britain, 1971–2005.

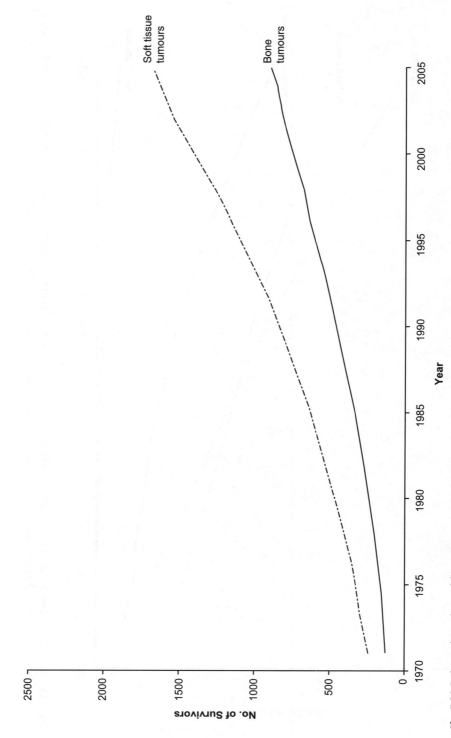

Fig. 5.30 Estimated numbers of five-year survivors of childhood malignant bone tumours and soft tissue sarcomas alive at the end of successive calendar years, by diagnostic group. Great Britain, 1971–2005.

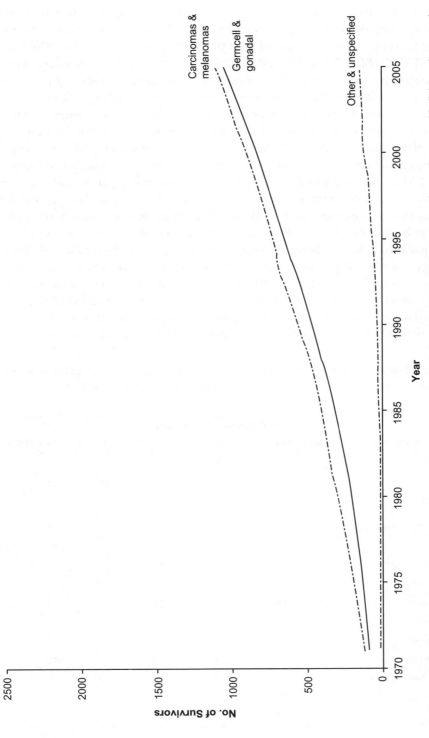

Fig. 5.31 Estimated numbers of five-year survivors of childhood germ cell, trophoblastic and gonadal tumours, other malignant epithelial neoplasms and malignant melanoma and other and unspecified malignant neoplasms alive at the end of successive calendar years, by diagnostic group. Great Britain, 1971–2005.

The British Childhood Cancer Survivor Study (BCCSS) was set up more recently, based on a cohort of nearly 16,000 survivors who had been diagnosed with cancer before the age of 15 years up to 1991, ascertained from the NRCT (Taylor *et al.*, 2004). The main ways in which the BCCSS differs from the CCSS are that it is population-based, survivors of retinoblastoma are included and maximum age at diagnosis is lower. At the time of this writing, data from the BCCSS are being analysed and prepared for publication.

A detailed account of the long-term health of survivors of childhood cancer is outside the scope of this book. Some mention should be made, however, of one of the most serious sequelae, namely, the development of a subsequent malignancy. Childhood cancer cases in the NRCT are followed up for occurrence of multiple neoplasms from a range of sources. The main ones are routine childhood cancer notifications to the NRCT, cancer registrations and death certificates received as a result of the flagging of survivors in the NHS Central Registers, responses to questionnaires within the BCCSS, and notifications from members of the UKCCSG. Formerly, multiple-tumour diagnoses were validated when possible by central pathological review, but this is now done by obtaining copies of pathology and other diagnostic reports. Table 5.23 shows the numbers of persons with childhood cancer diagnosed during 1951–2000, who also developed a subsequent cancer at any age during the same period, categorized according to calendar period of diagnosis of the first cancer and its diagnostic group. Table 5.24 shows the numbers of subsequent (second or later) cancers by period of diagnosis of the first cancer and diagnostic group

Table 5.23 Childhood cancer patients diagnosed during 1951–2000 who also had a subsequent cancer diagnosed during the same period, by type of first cancer and period of first cancer diagnosis

Diagnostic category of first cancer	Year of diagnosis of first cancer				
	1951–60	1961–70	1971–80	1981–90	1991–2000
All cancers	129	198	315	178	87
Leukaemia	0	11	76	50	21
Lymphoma	25	26	74	34	8
Hodgkin	15	22	51	16	3
Other and unspecified	10	4	23	18	5
CNS	43	53	73	39	28
Neuroblastoma, etc.	10	16	4	6	3
Retinoblastoma	22	38	15	10	3
Renal tumours	14	20	23	6	4
Hepatic tumours	0	1	0	0	1
Bone tumours	4	10	11	8	2
Soft tissue sarcomas	7	11	20	12	10
Germ cell and gonadal	1	3	6	8	3
Epithelial	3	8	13	4	3
Other	0	1	0	1	1

Table 5.24 Subsequent cancers diagnosed during 1951–2000 among patients who originally had childhood cancer diagnosed during the same period, by type of subsequent cancer and period of first cancer diagnosis

Diagnostic category of subsequent cancer	Year of diagnosis of first cancer				
	1951–60	1961–70	1971–80	1981–90	1991–2000
All cancers	137	204	330	181	89
Leukaemia	4	5	27	30	34
Lymphoma	2	6	16	14	4
CNS	24	42	86	49	19
Bone tumours	8	19	41	20	5
Soft tissue sarcomas	15	28	26	12	8
Germ cell tumours	0	1	5	0	1
Malignant melanoma	2	7	11	4	2
Carcinoma	77	92	107	44	9
Head and neck	4	8	7	8	1
Digestive	14	9	14	8	1
Lung	5	1	1	0	0
Skin	26	39	47	10	5
Breast	12	17	13	4	0
Female reproductive tract	2	3	5	0	0
Urinary	7	4	4	4	0
Thyroid	6	7	13	7	1
Other and unspecified	1	4	3	3	1
Other and unspecified	5	4	11	8	7

of the second cancer. The total numbers are larger than in Table 5.23 because they include 34 cases of third or later cancers. Table 5.25 shows the numbers of subsequent cancers according to diagnostic group of the first cancer. Among the first cancers, 26% were CNS tumours, 17% each were leukaemias and lymphomas, 10% were retinoblastomas, and 7% each were renal tumours and soft tissue sarcomas. Carcinomas accounted for 35% of subsequent cancers; of these, 39% were in the skin, 14% each in the digestive tract and breast and 10% in the thyroid. The most frequent other subsequent cancers were CNS tumours (23% of the total), leukaemia (11%) and sarcomas of bone and soft tissue (each 9–10%). The most frequent combinations of first and subsequent cancers were: CNS tumour followed by another CNS tumour; leukaemia followed by CNS tumour; retinoblastoma followed by bone tumour; CNS tumour, lymphoma and leukaemia followed by skin carcinoma; and leukaemia followed by another leukaemia. Among the much smaller number of multiple primary tumours occurring up to 1981, the most frequent combination was of retinoblastoma followed by osteosarcoma (Kingston et al., 1987). This reflected the already relatively large pool of survivors of retinoblastoma, a tumour that for many years had had a very high survival rate. The relative frequencies of first and subsequent cancers and combinations thereof will all be expected to continue to change with increasing follow-up. The high frequency of skin carcinoma, predominantly basal cell carcinoma, following

Table 5.25 Subsequent cancers diagnosed during 1951–2000 among patients who originally had childhood cancer diagnosed during the same period, by type of first cancer and subsequent cancer

Type of cancer	Diagnostic category of first cancer												
	Total	Leukaemia	Lymphoma	CNS	Neuroblastoma, etc.	Retino-blastoma	Renal	Hepatic	Bone	Soft tissue	Germ cell and gonadal	Epithelial	Other
Total	941	164	174	247	40	90	65	2	34	60	27	35	3
Leukaemia	100	28	24	17	6	5	3	2	2	3	8	2	0
Lymphoma	42	11	13	8	1	1	2	0	2	1	1	2	0
CNS	220	56	19	110	3	11	5	0	2	9	2	2	1
Bone	93	4	11	9	1	33	6	0	10	11	3	5	0
Soft tissue	89	3	12	16	9	23	8	0	6	5	1	6	0
Germ cell	7	0	1	3	0	0	1	0	0	0	2	0	0
Malignant melanoma	26	3	7	1	1	4	0	0	1	3	2	4	0
Carcinoma	329	51	84	73	16	11	37	0	11	24	8	13	1
Head and neck	28	8	6	5	1	1	1	0	1	2	1	1	1
Digestive	46	3	12	12	1	2	6	0	2	5	2	1	0
Lung	7	0	2	1	0	1	0	0	0	0	1	2	0

Skin	127	29	30	31	9	1	19	0	0	3	0	5	0
Breast	46	5	14	9	1	3	3	0	5	3	1	2	0
Female reproductive tract	10	0	1	4	0	0	0	0	0	3	0	2	0
Urinary	19	1	4	0	2	1	4	0	1	4	2	0	0
Thyroid	34	5	14	8	1	2	2	0	1	1	0	0	0
Other and unspecified	12	0	1	3	1	0	2	0	1	3	1	0	0
Other and unspecified	35	8	3	10	3	2	3	0	0	4	0	1	1

childhood leukaemia, lymphomas and CNS tumours has also been found in the American CCSS (Perkins *et al.*, 2005). Calculations of the risk of second malignant neoplasms are outside the scope of this book. Among three-year survivors diagnosed up to the end of 1987, there was a 4.2% cumulative risk of developing a second cancer during the next 25 years, giving a standardized incidence ratio of 6.2 (Jenkinson *et al.*, 2004); these risks were comparable with those in other population-based studies.

5.4 Conclusion

The past decades have seen dramatic improvements in the outcome for children diagnosed with cancer, resulting in an increasing proportion of survivors. For many childhood cancers, the aim is now to maintain the already high survival rates while refining treatment in order to reduce the frequency and severity of late effects. There are still some childhood cancers with much lower survival. In the 1990s, five-year survival was still below 50% for the diagnostic categories shown in Table 5.26. Together, they accounted for 203 registrations per year, 14% of the annual average of 1462 cases of all childhood cancers combined. CNS tumours, mostly gliomas and embryonal tumours, comprised one-half of the total and neuroblastoma accounted for slightly under one-third. The remainder were a miscellaneous collection of rare entities. Improving the outlook for these poor-prognosis diseases remains a challenge for paediatric oncology in the early twenty-first century.

Table 5.26 Categories of childhood cancer for which five-year survival of patients diagnosed during 1991–2000 was below 50%, along with number of cases (N) diagnosed during the same period

Diagnostic category	N
ALL (infants)	128
JMML/CMML	55
Choroid plexus carcinoma	40
Astrocytoma grade 3–4	238
Medulloblastoma (age 0–4 years)	185
PNET (except medulloblastoma)	161
ATRT	24
Unspecified glioma	328
Neuroblastoma (age 1–14 years)	629
Rhabdoid renal tumour	24
Hepatic carcinoma	25
Alveolar rhabdomyosarcoma	123
Extrarenal rhabdoid tumour	19
Colorectal carcinoma	11
DSRCT	12
Melanoma of CNS	9

Chapter 6

Childhood Cancer Mortality

KJ Bunch and CA Stiller

In this chapter, we describe in detail childhood cancer mortality in Britain during the period 1995–2004. Numbers of deaths and mortality rates are presented for the diagnostic groups and subgroups of ICCC-3 by age group and sex. Mortality data are also presented for five-yearly periods from 1965 to 2004 to give an indication of the trend in childhood cancer mortality over this period. Details of the methods and diagnostic groups included in the analyses that follow can be found in Chapter 2.

The deaths detailed in this chapter are those occurring before age 15 among children registered in the National Registry of Childhood Tumours (NRCT) and differ from childhood cancer mortality figures presented by the Office for National Statistics (ONS) and its predecessor, the Office of Population Censuses and Surveys (OPCS). In particular, ONS reports deaths occurring in England and Wales, whereas we also include deaths occurring in Scotland. More generally, in the vast majority of cases, the deaths described in this chapter are either the direct result of the child's cancer diagnosis or treatment related (Robertson *et al.*, 1992). However, the number of childhood cancer deaths reported will include a very small number unrelated to the child's earlier cancer diagnosis. Additionally, children diagnosed with cancer and registered in the NRCT who died after their fifteenth birthday would not be included among the deaths tabulated in this chapter.

6.1 Mortality rates 1995–2004

Table 6.1 shows the number of deaths among children with cancer during the period 1995–2004. A total of 3561 deaths were recorded, representing an overall age-standardized rate of 33.23 per million child years. Overall childhood cancer mortality rates were highest for children aged 1–4 at 35.98 per million child years and lowest for infants aged 0 at 29.58 per million child years. Death rates were higher for boys than girls, giving a sex ratio of 1.22 (the ratio of the mortality rate for boys, 36.44 per million child years, to that for girls, 29.86 per million child years). The largest numbers of deaths occurred among children diagnosed with central nervous system (CNS) or other brain tumours (1115) and leukaemia and related disorders (1099), with corresponding mortality rates of 10.47 and 10.12 per million child years, respectively. Of the remaining deaths, neuroblastoma and other peripheral nervous system tumours accounted for 378, soft tissue and extraosseous sarcomas 317, lymphomas 179, malignant bone tumours 169 and renal tumours 129, with fewer than 100 deaths in each of the remaining five diagnostic groups. The sex ratio varied among diagnostic groups, but was greater than 1 for the majority.

Text starts on page 210

Table 6.1 Childhood cancer mortality, numbers of deaths and rates, 1995–2004

ICCC-3	Numbers of deaths							Rates per million children				ASR		
	Age 0	Age 1–4	Age 5–9	Age 10–14	Total	Male	Female	Age 0	Age 1–4	Age 5–9	Age 10–14	Overall	Male	Female
Leukaemias, myeloproliferative and myelodysplastic diseases	54	277	370	398	1099	632	467	7.99	9.98	10.12	10.85	10.12	11.29	8.90
Lymphoid leukaemias	19	145	279	270	713	422	291	2.81	5.22	7.63	7.36	6.43	7.38	5.44
Acute myeloid leukaemias	23	86	60	95	264	143	121	3.40	3.10	1.64	2.59	2.50	2.63	2.37
Chronic myeloproliferative diseases	1	3	0	19	23	13	10	0.15	0.11	0.00	0.52	0.20	0.22	0.17
Myelodysplastic syndrome and other myeloproliferative diseases	7	37	26	9	79	42	37	1.04	1.33	0.71	0.25	0.79	0.82	0.76
Unspecified and other specified leukaemias	4	6	5	5	20	12	8	0.59	0.22	0.14	0.14	0.20	0.23	0.16
Lymphomas and reticuloendothelial neoplasms	4	32	67	76	179	123	56	0.59	1.15	1.83	2.07	1.60	2.12	1.05
Hodgkin lymphomas	0	0	4	10	14	10	4	0.00	0.00	0.11	0.27	0.11	0.16	0.06
Non-Hodgkin lymphomas (except Burkitt lymphoma)	2	24	46	51	123	85	38	0.30	0.86	1.26	1.39	1.10	1.48	0.71
Burkitt lymphoma	0	6	15	13	34	23	11	0.00	0.22	0.41	0.35	0.30	0.40	0.20
Miscellaneous lymphoreticular neoplasms	2	1	0	1	4	2	2	0.30	0.04	0.00	0.03	0.04	0.04	0.05
Unspecified lymphomas	0	1	2	1	4	3	1	0.00	0.04	0.05	0.03	0.04	0.05	0.02
CNS and miscellaneous intracranial and intraspinal neoplasms	69	316	418	312	1115	605	510	10.20	11.38	11.43	8.50	10.47	11.15	9.76
Ependymomas and choroid plexus tumour	9	57	43	21	130	79	51	1.33	2.05	1.18	0.57	1.28	1.53	1.03

Astrocytomas	14	47	130	141	332	166	166	2.07	1.69	3.56	3.84	2.95	2.91	2.98
Intracranial and intraspinal embryonal tumours	24	135	87	68	314	188	126	3.55	4.86	2.38	1.85	3.09	3.56	2.59
Other gliomas	2	43	130	54	229	114	115	0.30	1.55	3.56	1.47	2.08	2.03	2.13
Other specified intracranial and intraspinal neoplasms	2	15	15	17	49	24	25	0.30	0.54	0.41	0.46	0.46	0.44	0.47
Unspecified intracranial	18	19	13	11	61	34	27	2.66	0.68	0.36	0.30	0.62	0.68	0.56
Neuroblastoma and other peripheral nervous cell tumours	**14**	**188**	**137**	**39**	**378**	**237**	**141**	**2.07**	**6.77**	**3.75**	**1.06**	**3.77**	**4.62**	**2.89**
Neuroblastoma and ganglioneuroblastoma	14	188	135	37	374	235	139	2.07	6.77	3.69	1.01	3.74	4.58	2.86
Other peripheral nervous cell tumours	0	0	2	2	4	2	2	0.00	0.00	0.05	0.05	0.03	0.03	0.03
Retinoblastoma	**1**	**11**	**4**	**5**	**21**	**11**	**10**	**0.15**	**0.40**	**0.11**	**0.14**	**0.21**	**0.21**	**0.21**
Renal tumours	**10**	**52**	**45**	**22**	**129**	**65**	**64**	**1.48**	**1.87**	**1.23**	**0.60**	**1.27**	**1.26**	**1.27**
Nephroblastoma and other nonepithelial renal tumours	10	52	45	20	127	63	64	1.48	1.87	1.23	0.55	1.25	1.23	1.27
Renal carcinomas	0	0	0	2	2	2	0	0.00	0.00	0.00	0.05	0.02	0.03	0.00
Hepatic tumours	**6**	**24**	**3**	**17**	**50**	**30**	**20**	**0.89**	**0.86**	**0.08**	**0.46**	**0.50**	**0.61**	**0.38**
Hepatoblastoma	5	19	2	4	30	20	10	0.74	0.68	0.05	0.11	0.32	0.42	0.21
Hepatic carcinomas	1	4	1	13	19	9	10	0.15	0.14	0.03	0.35	0.17	0.17	0.17
Unspecified malignant hepatic tumours	0	1	0	0	1	1	0	0.00	0.04	0.00	0.00	0.01	0.02	0.00
Malignant bone tumours	**0**	**6**	**39**	**124**	**169**	**75**	**94**	**0.00**	**0.22**	**1.07**	**3.38**	**1.39**	**1.20**	**1.60**
Osteosarcomas	0	1	27	76	104	48	56	0.00	0.04	0.74	2.07	0.85	0.77	0.94
Chondrosarcomas	0	0	0	1	1	0	1	0.00	0.00	0.00	0.03	0.01	0.00	0.02

Table 6.1 (continued) Childhood cancer mortality, numbers of deaths and rates, 1995–2004

Ewing tumour and related bone sarcomas	0	5	12	45	62	27	35	0.00	0.18	0.33	1.23	0.52	0.43	0.61
Other specified malignant bone tumours	0	0	0	2	2	0	2	0.00	0.00	0.00	0.05	0.02	0.00	0.03
Soft tissue and other extraosseous sarcomas	**26**	**71**	**107**	**113**	**317**	**174**	**143**	**3.84**	**2.56**	**2.93**	**3.08**	**2.93**	**3.14**	**2.71**
Rhabdomyosarcomas	3	48	67	53	171	92	79	0.44	1.73	1.83	1.44	1.58	1.67	1.48
Fibrosarcomas, peripheral nerve sheath tumours and other fibrous neoplasms	2	3	3	9	17	15	2	0.30	0.11	0.08	0.25	0.15	0.26	0.05
Kaposi sarcoma	0	0	2	1	3	0	3	0.00	0.00	0.05	0.03	0.03	0.00	0.05
Other specified soft tissue sarcomas	11	17	25	42	95	53	42	1.63	0.61	0.68	1.14	0.87	0.94	0.79
Unspecified soft tissue sarcomas	10	3	10	8	31	14	17	1.48	0.11	0.27	0.22	0.30	0.27	0.33
Germ cell tumours, trophoblastic tumours and neoplasms of gonads	**12**	**12**	**7**	**13**	**44**	**15**	**29**	**1.77**	**0.43**	**0.19**	**0.35**	**0.44**	**0.29**	**0.59**
Intracranial and intraspinal germ cell	5	3	6	6	20	8	12	0.74	0.11	0.16	0.16	0.19	0.14	0.25
Malignant extracranial and extra-gonadal germ cell tumours	7	8	1	3	19	6	13	1.04	0.29	0.03	0.08	0.20	0.13	0.28
Malignant gonadal germ cell tumours	0	1	0	2	3	1	2	0.00	0.04	0.00	0.05	0.03	0.02	0.03
Gonadal carcinomas	0	0	0	2	2	0	2	0.00	0.00	0.00	0.05	0.02	0.00	0.03
Other malignant epithelial neoplasms and malignant melanomas	**3**	**7**	**15**	**24**	**49**	**27**	**22**	**0.44**	**0.25**	**0.41**	**0.65**	**0.43**	**0.47**	**0.40**

Adrenocortical carcinomas	0	3	6	2	11	4	7	0.00	0.11	0.16	0.05	0.10	0.07	0.13
Thyroid carcinomas	0	0	2	0	2	1	1	0.00	0.00	0.05	0.00	0.02	0.02	0.02
Nasopharyngeal carcinomas	0	0	0	2	2	1	1	0.00	0.00	0.00	0.05	0.02	0.02	0.02
Malignant melanomas	2	4	4	7	17	12	5	0.30	0.14	0.11	0.19	0.16	0.21	0.10
Skin carcinomas	0	0	0	0	0	0	0	0.00	0.00	0.00	0.00	0.00	0.00	0.00
Other and unspecified carcinomas	1	0	3	13	17	9	8	0.15	0.00	0.08	0.35	0.14	0.15	0.13
Other and unspecified malignant neoplasms	**1**	**3**	**0**	**7**	**11**	**5**	**6**	**0.15**	**0.11**	**0.00**	**0.19**	**0.10**	**0.09**	**0.11**
Other specified malignant tumours	0	2	0	4	6	2	4	0.00	0.07	0.00	0.11	0.05	0.04	0.07
Other unspecified malignant tumours	1	1	0	3	5	3	2	0.15	0.04	0.00	0.08	0.05	0.05	0.04
Total	200	999	1212	1150	3561	1999	1562	29.58	35.98	33.15	31.35	33.23	36.44	29.86

The increased mortality rates for boys were most marked for lymphomas, hepatic tumours and neuroblastoma (sex ratios 2.02, 1.61 and 1.60, respectively). Bone tumours were a notable exception to the general pattern, with a mortality rate for girls of 1.60 per million child years compared to 1.20 for boys (sex ratio 0.75). The pattern of mortality rates by death age group also varied among the different diagnostic groups. The mortality rate for leukaemias was lowest in infants, 7.99 per million child years, rising to 9.98 and 10.12 per million child years in children aged 1–4 and 5–9, respectively, and rising further to 10.85 per million child years in those aged 10–14 years. For CNS tumours, the mortality rate was lower in the oldest children, while for bone tumours, few deaths occurred in children under 10 years of age. Clearly, the age distribution of deaths for the individual diagnostic groups will, to a large extent, be determined by the age distribution of incidence for that group.

The different diagnostic groups and subgroups made different contributions to total age-standardized mortality and incidence. Whereas leukaemias accounted for 33% of the age-standardized incidence rate in 1991–2000 (Table 3.2), only 30% of the age-standardized mortality rate was attributable to leukaemias. This difference reflects the fact that the survival rate for leukaemia is higher than that for childhood cancer overall. Lymphoid leukaemia, which has a high survival rate (five-year survival 82% in 1991–2000, Table 5.1), accounted for 26% of childhood cancer incidence, but only 19% of mortality. In contrast, acute myeloid leukaemia, which has a lower survival rate (five-year survival rate 58% in 1991–2000, Table 5.1), was responsible for 4.8% of childhood cancer incidence but 7.5% of mortality. Both CNS tumours and neuroblastoma contributed relatively more to childhood cancer mortality than to incidence (32% versus 24% and 11% versus 7%, respectively), whereas lymphomas, renal tumours and retinoblastoma were each responsible for a smaller proportion of childhood cancer mortality than incidence (5% versus 9%, 4% versus 6% and 1% versus 3%, respectively).

An additional factor that influences the balance between the incidence and mortality contributions of the different diagnostic groups is the age at diagnosis. Survival to 5 years beyond diagnosis is a generally accepted marker of successful treatment. For a given five-year survival rate, children diagnosed at a younger age will be more likely to die before reaching age 15 (and thus contribute to the mortality data described here) than children diagnosed at an older age.

Overall cancer incidence rates were higher in infants and children aged 1–4 (188.33 and 185.55 per million child years, respectively, in 1991–2000, Table 3.2) than in older children (108.15 and 110.01 per million child years for children aged 5–9 and 10–14, respectively, Table 3.2). In contrast, the variation in mortality rates across the age groups was less marked. Nevertheless, mortality was lowest in infants (29.58 per million child years), reached a peak in children aged 1–4 (35.98 per million child years) and then fell to 33.15 and 31.35 per million child years in children aged 5–9 and 10–14, respectively. This difference in age distribution is accounted for by children dying at varying lengths of time after diagnosis and by variations in prognosis with age for many types of cancer. For neuroblastoma, in which the majority of cases occur in infants (Table 3.2), the mortality rate was, however, highest in children aged 1–4 as a result of the much lower survival rate for this age group (five-year survival rates for 1991–2000: 83% for infants and 46% for children aged 1–4; see Table 5.3).

Direct comparisons between the detailed cancer mortality rates for the period 1995–2004 reported here and rates for other countries are difficult, as no studies have reported on the same time period. The most recent comparative international mortality data available are those in the International Agency for Research on Cancer's GLOBOCAN 2002 database (Ferlay *et al.*, 2004). Mortality data in this database are sourced from different national agencies and represent deaths in a single year or, in some cases, the average over a small number of years. Regional figures are derived by calculating population-weighted averages of the values for the different countries within the region. The death rates presented here differ from the GLOBOCAN rates for ages 0–14 in the United Kingdom: we report mortality rates of 36.44 and 29.86 per million child years for boys and girls, respectively, whereas GLOBOCAN gives rates of 34.40 (boys) and 26.10 (girls) per million child years for all cancer sites except skin, based on deaths reported for 1999. Inevitably, there is some year-to-year random variation in the numbers of childhood cancer deaths and, given the small numbers involved, this can result in apparently dramatic variation in corresponding mortality rates. While GLOBOCAN enables crude comparisons of the burden of cancer mortality in different countries and regions of the world, the mortality rates we present, which are based on deaths over a ten-year period, represent a better estimate of the true childhood cancer mortality rate for England, Wales and Scotland than any single year's figures.

GLOBOCAN groups the United Kingdom with Eire, the Nordic countries (Denmark, Finland, Iceland, Norway and Sweden) and the Baltic states (Latvia, Lithuania and Estonia) to form a Northern European region. Within this region, the childhood mortality rates for the Baltic countries and Iceland are the highest and those for the other Nordic countries and Eire are the lowest. However, it must be noted that rates given for Iceland and Eire are based on only 2 and 17 deaths, respectively, compared to 334 childhood cancer deaths reported in the United Kingdom. Whether considering our data based on 1995–2004 deaths or GLOBOCAN data based on 1999 figures, the United Kingdom childhood mortality rates sit between the two extremes described above (Table 6.2). Comparing Northern Europe with other more developed regions, childhood cancer mortality rates are lower in the United States, Canada, Western Europe and Japan; higher in Australia/New Zealand and Southern Europe; and considerably higher in Eastern Europe. Within GLOBOCAN, mortality is stratified by cancer site based on the sites contributing most to adult rather than childhood mortality, thus limiting the number of meaningful comparisons that can be made. Childhood leukaemia mortality rates show similar regional variations to childhood cancer overall. However, for brain and nervous system tumours, while childhood mortality rates are lowest in Japan, the United States, Canada and Western Europe and highest in Eastern Europe, rates for Northern Europe are similar to those for Australia/New Zealand and higher than those for Southern Europe. For all other sites combined (including lymphomas and non-CNS solid tumours), childhood mortality rates are lowest in Japan, Canada, the United States, Northern and Western Europe; slightly higher in Southern Europe and Australia/New Zealand and considerably higher in Eastern Europe.

Table 6.2 International childhood cancer mortality rates from GLOBOCAN 2002 with comparative rates for NRCT data (1995–2004)

	All sites except skin (Deaths per million child years)		Leukaemia		Brain and nervous system		Other sites*	
	Male	Female	Male	Female	Male	Female	Male	Female
Northern Europe	33.3	26.0	10.9	9.7	10.4	8.2	12.0	8.1
United Kingdom	34.4	26.1	12.0	10.8	11.3	8.1	11.1	7.2
Eire	25.9	14.9	7.0	5.0	2.3	2.5	16.6	7.4
Nordic countries	27.1	24.5	7.9	7.5	8.4	7.9	10.8	9.1
Baltic states	49.7	37.4	14.9	10.4	14.0	13.3	20.8	13.7
Western Europe	30.9	22.1	9.9	6.3	9.9	6.5	11.1	9.3
Southern Europe	34.7	30.4	12.3	10.3	9.8	6.9	12.6	13.2
Eastern Europe	55.3	45.6	17.6	13.8	13.8	12.3	23.9	19.5
USA	26.8	22.9	8.6	7.0	7.5	7.0	10.7	8.9
Canada	23.9	26.2	8.5	7.6	6.9	8.6	8.5	10.0
Australia/New Zealand	37.0	26.7	12.2	10.1	12.4	6.0	12.4	10.6
Japan	27.6	18.5	11.5	8.2	5.1	3.5	11.0	6.8
NRCT (1995–2004 deaths)	36.44	29.86	11.29	8.90	11.15	9.76	14.00	11.20

* Rates for other sites may be subject to small rounding errors.

6.2 **Mortality trends**

Trends in overall childhood cancer mortality during the 40-year period 1965–2004 are shown in Table 6.3, Figures 6.1 and 6.2. Considering all age groups together, mortality rates in 2000–2004 were less than half those of 1965–1969. These trends in mortality reduction were broadly similar for both boys and girls (Fig. 6.1). Mortality rates fell during the period 1965–2004 for all age groups (Fig. 6.2). For infants, there was a considerable decrease in mortality between 1995–1999 and 2000–2004, while for the older age groups, mortality rates appeared to be stabilizing.

Mortality trends for the individual diagnostic groups are shown in Tables 6.4–6.15 and Figs. 6.3–6.14.

Mortality rates among children diagnosed with leukaemia fell throughout the period 1965–2004 (Table 6.4 and Fig. 6.3), with the most marked decrease in mortality occurring in the earlier years of the period. Considering the leukaemia mortality rates for the different age groups (Fig. 6.6), the decrease during this period was greatest for children aged 1–4 and least marked for the oldest age group (children aged 10–14 years). Mortality rates in children with a CNS tumour decreased from 15.51 per million child years in 1965–1969 to 9.93 per million child years in 2000–2004 (Table 6.6 and Fig. 6.3). Mortality rates among boys with CNS tumours were higher than those in girls throughout the study period (Fig. 6.7); however, by 2000–2004 the sex ratio was 1.05, compared to 1.24 at the start of the study period. In contrast, mortality rates in children with lymphoma were relatively low at the beginning of the study period (6.67 per million child years) and had fallen to 1.61 per million child years by 2000–2004, with the reduction in mortality occurring largely in the earlier years of the study period (Table 6.5 and Fig. 6.3).

Mortality rates in children with neuroblastoma and associated peripheral nervous system tumours were 7.32 per million child years in 1965–1969, decreased over the following 20 years and then remained relatively constant during the remainder of the study period (Table 6.7 and Fig. 6.3). Mortality rates for the different age groups, however, showed considerable variation. Neuroblastoma mortality rates in infants and children aged 1–4 have fallen considerably during the study period (Fig. 6.8), while death rates in the two older age groups have remained much more constant. Mortality rates for boys with neuroblastoma were higher than those of girls at the start of the study period (sex ratio 1.16 in 1965–1969) (Fig. 6.9). By 1980–1984, the two mortality rates were the same but then after 1985, the mortality rate in girls fell more rapidly than that in boys, so that by 2000–2004 the sex ratio had risen to 1.68.

Deaths in children with retinoblastoma have been rare throughout the study period but the overall mortality rate has nevertheless fallen from 0.55 per million child years in 1965–1969 to 0.15 in 2000–2004 (Table 6.8 and Fig. 6.4). The overall mortality rate in children with renal tumours fell from 4.91 per million child years in 1965–1969 to 1.35 per million child years in 1985–1989 and has remained relatively constant during the remainder of the study period (Table 6.9 and Fig. 6.4). The early decrease in mortality rates for this diagnostic group was largely confined to infants and children aged 1–4 (Fig. 6.10). The overall mortality in children with hepatic tumours were low (rates of less than

Text starts on page 233

Table 6.3 Trends in childhood cancer mortality

Death period	Numbers of deaths							Rates per million children				ASR		
	Age 0	Age 1–4	Age 5–9	Age 10–14	Persons	Male	Female	Age 0	Age 1–4	Age 5–9	Age 10–14	Persons	Male	Female
1965–1969	290	1782	1480	1142	4694	2657	2037	63.30	96.54	70.23	60.82	75.11	82.88	66.93
1970–1974	245	1412	1523	1135	4315	2474	1841	61.15	81.84	67.33	54.07	67.50	75.25	59.33
1975–1979	173	913	1302	1136	3524	2083	1441	53.00	65.14	62.09	50.25	58.90	67.63	49.68
1980–1984	155	766	839	957	2717	1506	1211	44.68	57.10	49.02	45.83	50.26	54.18	46.13
1985–1989	145	664	678	640	2127	1145	982	39.64	47.04	39.97	37.23	41.34	43.22	39.35
1990–1994	131	571	719	617	2038	1149	889	35.06	38.26	40.19	36.23	38.05	41.92	34.00
1995–1999	122	510	664	558	1854	1058	796	35.02	35.40	35.50	31.11	34.16	38.11	30.02
2000–2004	74	472	534	584	1664	924	740	22.57	35.33	29.91	31.14	31.38	34.01	28.61

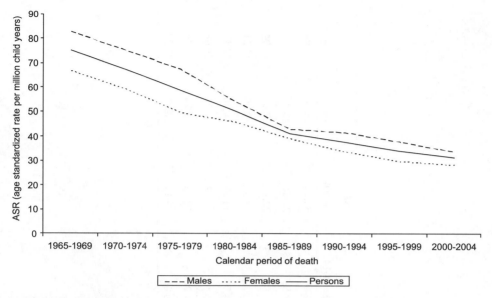

Fig. 6.1 Deaths before age 15 of children diagnosed with a malignant neoplasm.

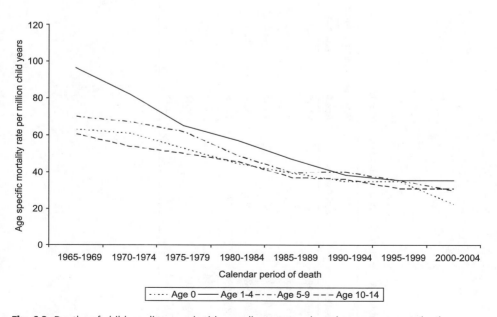

Fig. 6.2 Deaths of children diagnosed with a malignant neoplasm by age group at death.

Table 6.4 Trends in childhood leukaemia mortality

Death Period	Total Deaths	Rates per million children					ASR		
		Age 0	Age 1–4	Age 5–9	Age 10–14	Persons	Male	Female
1965–1969	1883	17.46	39.82	30.46	22.69	30.10	33.00	27.04
1970–1974	1703	20.22	31.65	30.37	18.53	26.54	29.24	23.71
1975–1979	1389	16.85	22.98	27.95	18.85	22.91	27.61	17.94
1980–1984	1006	13.84	19.53	20.27	16.72	18.51	20.69	16.21
1985–1989	703	11.48	14.73	12.44	14.08	13.55	14.86	12.17
1990–1994	603	13.11	9.78	12.24	11.10	11.22	13.26	9.08
1995–1999	568	9.47	8.75	11.07	11.26	10.28	11.74	8.76
2000–2004	488	5.18	10.03	8.34	10.03	9.11	10.17	7.99

Table 6.5 Trends in childhood lymphoma mortality

Death period	Total deaths	Rates per million children					ASR		
		Age 0	Age 1–4	Age 5–9	Age 10–14	Persons	Male	Female
1965–1969	424	2.84	4.98	7.59	8.47	6.67	9.22	3.98
1970–1974	365	1.25	4.81	6.01	6.72	5.48	7.65	3.19
1975–1979	290	0.61	3.00	5.06	6.19	4.40	5.95	2.78
1980–1984	190	2.31	2.31	3.56	4.31	3.30	4.33	2.20
1985–1989	112	0.55	1.56	2.30	2.85	2.09	2.83	1.32
1990–1994	93	0.54	1.27	1.84	2.29	1.70	2.25	1.12
1995–1999	90	0.86	0.90	1.98	2.06	1.58	2.16	0.98
2000–2004	89	0.30	1.42	1.68	2.08	1.61	2.08	1.12

Table 6.6 Trends in childhood CNS tumour mortality

Death period	Total deaths	Rates per million children					ASR		
		Age 0	Age 1–4	Age 5–9	Age 10–14		Persons	Male	Female
1965–1969	976	13.75	15.93	17.18	13.69		15.51	17.14	13.80
1970–1974	988	10.98	16.58	16.22	13.86		15.24	17.23	13.15
1975–1979	882	13.48	16.34	16.17	11.94		14.79	16.27	13.22
1980–1984	720	12.97	13.57	13.73	12.36		13.22	14.23	12.16
1985–1989	606	12.30	11.55	13.62	9.71		11.74	11.95	11.53
1990–1994	663	9.63	10.12	15.21	11.98		12.26	12.67	11.83
1995–1999	594	12.06	11.59	12.03	8.92		10.99	12.12	9.82
2000–2004	521	8.23	11.15	10.81	8.11		9.93	10.15	9.70

Table 6.7 Trends in childhood neuroblastoma and other peripheral nervous cell tumour mortality

Death period	Total deaths	Rates per million children					ASR		
		Age 0	Age 1–4	Age 5–9	Age 10–14		Persons	Male	Female
1965–1969	447	13.75	13.60	4.32	2.24		7.32	7.84	6.77
1970–1974	388	14.48	10.95	4.02	2.38		6.50	7.62	5.33
1975–1979	274	8.27	9.49	4.01	1.33		5.26	6.34	4.12
1980–1984	222	6.05	9.99	3.04	0.72		4.75	4.75	4.76
1985–1989	251	5.19	9.85	4.77	0.70		5.19	5.32	5.06
1990–1994	254	3.48	8.64	5.25	1.06		4.95	5.67	4.20
1995–1999	203	2.58	7.01	4.22	0.78		3.96	4.76	3.12
2000–2004	175	1.52	6.51	3.25	1.33		3.57	4.45	2.65

Table 6.8 Trends in childhood retinoblastoma mortality

Death period	Total deaths	Rates per million children					ASR		
		Age 0	Age 1–4	Age 5–9	Age 10–14		Persons	Male	Female
1965–1969	33	0.00	1.46	0.14	0.16		0.55	0.58	0.51
1970–1974	35	0.50	1.56	0.13	0.14		0.61	0.58	0.64
1975–1979	28	0.61	1.36	0.24	0.09		0.57	0.43	0.72
1980–1984	17	0.00	0.82	0.29	0.05		0.36	0.38	0.34
1985–1989	18	0.00	0.92	0.18	0.12		0.38	0.32	0.43
1990–1994	14	0.27	0.40	0.39	0.00		0.27	0.26	0.29
1995–1999	14	0.00	0.49	0.21	0.17		0.27	0.29	0.24
2000–2004	7	0.30	0.30	0.00	0.11		0.15	0.12	0.18

Table 6.9 Trends in childhood renal tumour mortality

| Death period | Total deaths | Rates per million children | | | | ASR | | |
		Age 0	Age 1–4	Age 5–9	Age 10–14	Persons	Male	Female
1965–1969	300	5.24	10.35	3.37	0.75	4.91	4.79	5.05
1970–1974	207	2.50	6.09	3.09	1.05	3.38	3.04	3.74
1975–1979	119	2.45	4.00	1.86	0.71	2.23	1.95	2.53
1980–1984	95	2.02	2.98	2.22	0.48	1.93	1.96	1.91
1985–1989	67	1.37	2.13	1.24	0.64	1.35	1.03	1.68
1990–1994	81	2.14	2.81	1.17	0.59	1.59	1.53	1.64
1995–1999	69	1.15	2.22	1.28	0.50	1.34	1.41	1.25
2000–2004	60	1.83	1.50	1.18	0.69	1.19	1.09	1.29

Table 6.10 Trends in childhood hepatic tumour mortality

Death period	Total deaths	Rates per million children					ASR		
		Age 0	Age 1–4	Age 5–9	Age 10–14	Persons	Male	Female
1965–1969	43	2.40	1.19	0.14	0.37	0.71	0.90	0.51
1970–1974	37	2.50	1.04	0.18	0.24	0.64	0.67	0.61
1975–1979	40	2.45	1.36	0.33	0.27	0.79	0.70	0.89
1980–1984	34	2.31	1.04	0.23	0.38	0.69	0.61	0.77
1985–1989	35	2.46	0.99	0.35	0.35	0.71	0.99	0.42
1990–1994	25	0.80	0.80	0.22	0.35	0.49	0.72	0.24
1995–1999	19	0.86	0.69	0.00	0.33	0.38	0.55	0.20
2000–2004	31	0.91	1.05	0.17	0.59	0.62	0.68	0.56

Table 6.11 Trends in childhood malignant bone tumour mortality

| Death period | Total deaths | Rates per million children | | | | | ASR | | |
		Age 0	Age 1–4	Age 5–9	Age 10–14		Persons	Male	Female
1965–1969	169	0.00	0.38	1.80	6.60		2.62	2.49	2.75
1970–1974	177	0.00	0.46	2.03	5.86		2.50	2.46	2.54
1975–1979	166	0.31	0.21	1.81	5.49		2.27	2.36	2.17
1980–1984	162	0.00	0.52	1.75	5.99		2.47	2.30	2.63
1985–1989	103	0.27	0.35	1.12	4.54		1.81	1.64	1.99
1990–1994	74	0.00	0.13	0.56	3.64		1.28	1.28	1.27
1995–1999	72	0.00	0.07	0.91	3.01		1.19	1.03	1.36
2000–2004	97	0.00	0.37	1.23	3.73		1.60	1.37	1.84

Table 6.12 Trends in childhood soft tissue sarcoma mortality

Death period	Total deaths	Rates per million children					ASR		
		Age 0	Age 1–4	Age 5–9	Age 10–14		Persons	Male	Female
1965–1969	225	2.62	4.71	3.37	2.93		3.60	3.95	3.23
1970–1974	260	6.24	5.10	3.98	2.72		4.13	4.54	3.71
1975–1979	201	4.29	3.64	3.29	2.96		3.38	3.97	2.76
1980–1984	163	2.31	3.95	2.86	2.54		3.06	3.30	2.81
1985–1989	159	3.28	3.97	3.12	2.21		3.13	2.98	3.30
1990–1994	168	3.21	3.28	2.63	3.52		3.14	3.08	3.19
1995–1999	168	5.74	2.78	3.15	2.73		3.12	3.34	2.88
2000–2004	149	1.83	2.32	2.69	3.41		2.72	2.92	2.50

Table 6.13 Trends in childhood germ cell and gonadal tumour mortality

| Death period | Total deaths | Rates per million children | | | | | ASR | | |
		Age 0	Age 1–4	Age 5–9	Age 10–14	Persons	Male	Female
1965–1969	94	3.06	2.38	0.76	1.07	1.53	1.25	1.82
1970–1974	94	1.50	2.72	0.62	1.29	1.53	1.24	1.84
1975–1979	77	2.45	2.21	0.72	1.02	1.40	1.20	1.61
1980–1984	63	2.31	1.79	0.29	1.25	1.19	0.93	1.46
1985–1989	42	2.46	0.71	0.41	0.93	0.81	0.74	0.89
1990–1994	37	1.61	0.74	0.39	0.76	0.70	0.74	0.66
1995–1999	29	2.01	0.62	0.32	0.39	0.57	0.30	0.84
2000–2004	15	1.52	0.22	0.06	0.32	0.30	0.28	0.32

Table 6.14 Trends in childhood carcinoma and melanoma mortality

Death period	Total deaths	Rates per million children					ASR		
		Age 0	Age 1–4	Age 5–9	Age 10–14		Persons	Male	Female
1965–1969	52	1.09	0.65	0.71	1.07		0.82	0.84	0.81
1970–1974	38	0.50	0.75	0.31	0.76		0.59	0.54	0.65
1975–1979	44	0.92	0.29	0.48	1.19		0.66	0.55	0.77
1980–1984	37	0.29	0.45	0.64	0.91		0.63	0.50	0.77
1985–1989	21	0.00	0.14	0.18	0.93		0.37	0.30	0.45
1990–1994	24	0.00	0.20	0.28	0.94		0.43	0.41	0.44
1995–1999	22	0.29	0.21	0.32	0.67		0.38	0.38	0.39
2000–2004	27	0.61	0.30	0.50	0.64		0.49	0.55	0.42

Table 6.15 Trends in childhood mortality in patients diagnosed with other and unspecified tumours

Death period	Total deaths	Rates per million children					ASR		
		Age 0	Age 1–4	Age 5–9	Age 10–14		Persons	Male	Female
1965–1969	48	1.09	1.08	0.38	0.80		0.77	0.87	0.67
1970–1974	23	0.50	0.12	0.35	0.52		0.34	0.45	0.23
1975–1979	14	0.31	0.29	0.19	0.22		0.24	0.31	0.16
1980–1984	8	0.29	0.15	0.12	0.14		0.15	0.20	0.10
1985–1989	10	0.27	0.14	0.24	0.17		0.19	0.27	0.11
1990–1994	2	0.27	0.07	0.00	0.00		0.04	0.04	0.04
1995–1999	6	0.00	0.07	0.00	0.28		0.10	0.03	0.18
2000–2004	5	0.30	0.15	0.00	0.11		0.10	0.15	0.05

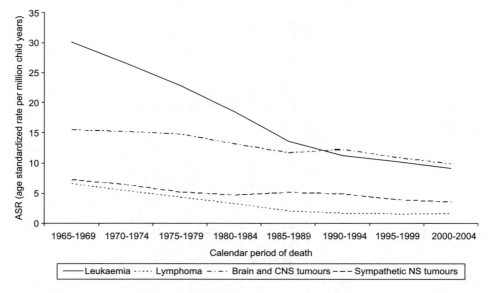

Fig. 6.3 Deaths before age 15 of children diagnosed with a malignant neoplasm. i. Leukaemia, lymphoma, central nervous system and sympathetic nervous system tumours.

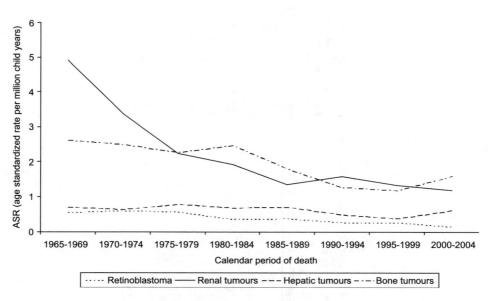

Fig. 6.4 Deaths before age 15 of children diagnosed with a malignant neoplasm. ii. Retinoblastoma, renal, hepatic and bone tumours.

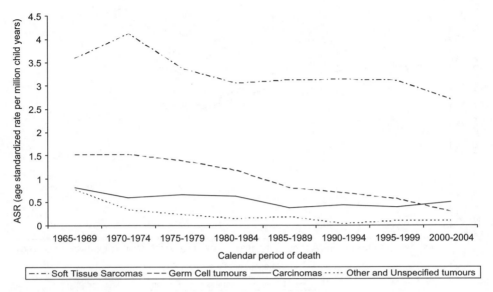

Fig. 6.5 Deaths before age 15 of children diagnosed with a malignant neoplasm. iii. Sarcomas, germ cell tumours, carcinomas and other and unspecified tumours.

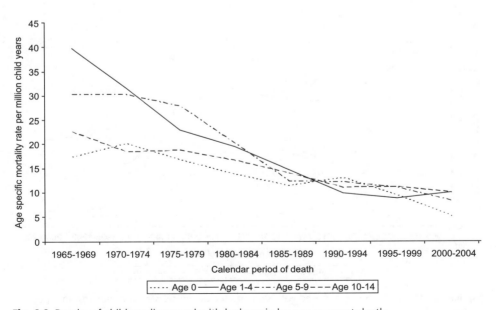

Fig. 6.6 Deaths of children diagnosed with leukaemia by age group at death.

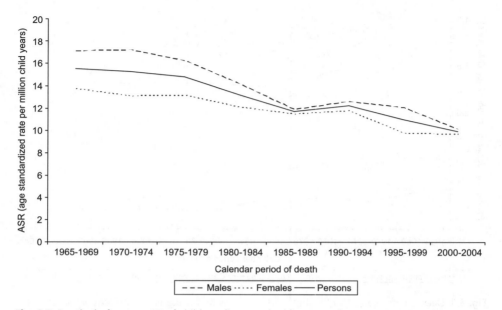

Fig. 6.7 Deaths before age 15 of children diagnosed with a central nervous system tumour by sex.

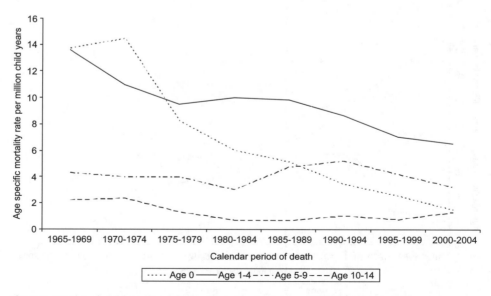

Fig. 6.8 Deaths of children diagnosed with sympathetic nervous system tumours by age group at death.

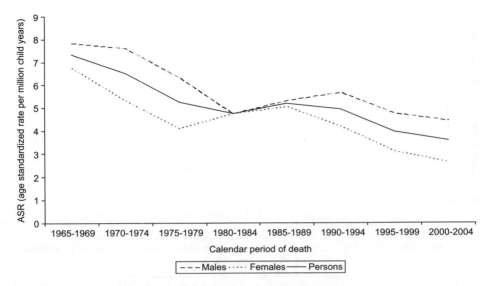

Fig. 6.9 Deaths before age 15 of children diagnosed with a sympathetic nervous system tumour by sex.

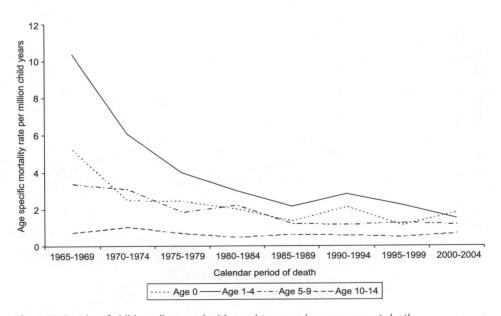

Fig. 6.10 Deaths of children diagnosed with renal tumours by age group at death.

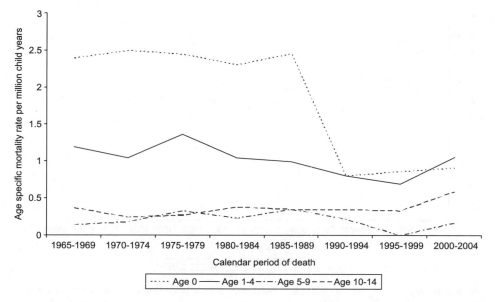

Fig. 6.11 Deaths of children diagnosed with hepatic tumours by age group at death.

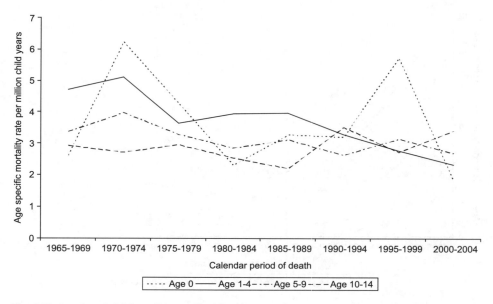

Fig. 6.12 Deaths of children diagnosed with soft tissue sarcomas by age group at death.

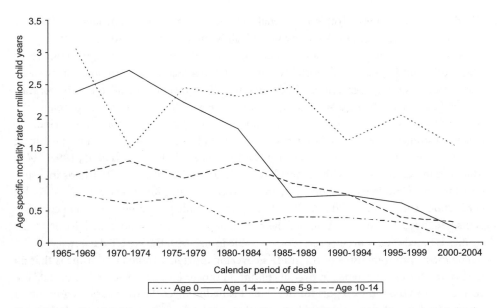

Fig. 6.13 Deaths of children diagnosed with germ cell and gonadal tumours by age group at death.

1 per million child years) throughout the study period, with no clear trend (Table 6.10 and Fig. 6.4). Considering the different age groups separately (Fig. 6.11), the mortality rate in infants with hepatic tumours fell sharply between 1985–1989 and 1990–1994, but then appeared to rise slightly over the following 10 years. Death rates in children with malignant bone tumours fell from 2.62 per million child years in 1965–1969 to 1.60 per million child years in 2000–2004 (Table 6.11 and Fig. 6.4).

The mortality rate in children with soft tissue sarcomas reached 4.13 per million child years during 1970–1974 but had fallen to 2.72 per million child years by 2000–2004 (Table 6.12 and Fig. 6.5). The mortality rate in infants with this diagnosis rose initially, then fell considerably before rising again in 1995–1999 then finally falling in 2000–2004 (Fig. 6.12). However, these fluctuations may well be due to chance, given the small numbers of infants involved. Mortality rates in children aged 1–4 tended to fall over the study period, while those in children aged 5–9 changed little and those in the oldest children, aged 10–14 showed a small increase over the study period. Children with germ cell and gonadal tumours had a mortality rate of 1.53 per million child years in 1965–1969, which had fallen to 0.30 per million child years by 2000–2004 (Table 6.13 and Fig. 6.5). The decrease was greatest in children aged 1–4 and 5–9 (Fig. 6.13). The mortality rates for infants with germ cell tumours varied during the study period but had decreased to 1.52 per million child years by 2000–2004. Mortality rates in children aged 5–9 and 10–14 were low throughout the study period, falling to 0.06 and 0.32 per million child years, respectively, by 2000–2004.

Children with carcinomas (other than renal, hepatic and gonadal) and melanomas had low mortality rates throughout the study period, showing only small reductions during the early part of the study period and remaining relatively constant during the later years (Table 6.14 and Fig. 6.5). The mortality rates in children diagnosed with other or unspecified tumours was 0.77 per million child years in 1965–1969 and had fallen to 0.10 per million child years by 2000–2004 (Table 6.15 and Fig. 6.5). This reduction was probably the result of more precise diagnostic classification during the later part of the study period.

Several studies have reported on trends in childhood cancer mortality in Europe during the second half of the twentieth century (La Vecchia *et al.*, 1991; Levi *et al.*, 1992, 2001; Martos and Olsen, 1993), while others have looked in detail at mortality trends in a specific European country or region (Levi and La Vecchia, 1988; Kunze *et al.*, 1997; Gonzalez *et al.*, 2004; Zuccolo *et al.*, 2004). These later studies, while providing interesting comparisons, are limited by the small size of the populations or regions concerned. None of the studies is based on a mortality series comparable in size with the NRCT dataset.

The most comprehensive of the studies covering mortality trends in Europe is that by Levi *et al.* (2001). The trends in overall childhood cancer mortality shown in our data are very similar to those they report for the United Kingdom over the time period common to the two studies, although it should be noted that the deaths Levi *et al.* report include those attributable to benign neoplasms of all sites, whereas our series includes only nonmalignant CNS tumours. The United Kingdom has shown decreases in overall childhood cancer mortality similar to those shown for most other Western European countries and appreciably greater than observed in Eastern Europe. The latest period for which Levi *et al.* report mortality is 1990–1994 and, like the comparisons made earlier in the chapter based on GLOBOCAN data, these figures show the highest mortality rates occurring in Eastern European countries. Among the trends for individual sites that are described in detail, our data show very similar mortality patterns for leukaemias, bone, eye and renal tumours, generally reflecting the trends for mortality reduction evident across Western Europe.

Childhood leukaemia mortality trends in Europe, Japan and the United States were compared by Levi *et al.* (2000) as part of a larger study of all-age leukaemia mortality over the period 1960–1997. Again, the reductions in leukaemia mortality demonstrated by the NRCT data are similar to those tabulated by Levi *et al.* for the countries of the European Union and more pronounced than those for Eastern Europe. The reduction in childhood leukaemia mortality in Japan was only slightly less than that in the European Union, although earlier mortality rates from Japan may have been affected by low diagnostic and certification accuracy (Levi *et al.*, 2000). The reduction in childhood leukaemia mortality rates is shown to be greater in the United States than in other more developed countries.

Mortality rates in children diagnosed with brain and central nervous system tumours (CNS) have fallen during the period of our study (36%), but less dramatically than those for several other diagnostic groups, e.g. leukaemia (70%), lymphomas (76%) and renal tumours (76%). Legler *et al.* (1999) report rather lower childhood brain tumour mortality rates in the United States for the period 1975–1995 than the NRCT data give for England, Wales and Scotland. There were also similar trends in childhood brain tumour mortality for that period, but the halt in the reduction in mortality rates observed in our data between 1985–89 and 1990–94 (Fig. 6.7) occurred a few years earlier in the United States. Changes in the histological classification of brain tumours, developments in neurosurgical practice and increasing availability of magnetic resonance imaging may all have contributed to this feature of the trend in childhood brain tumour mortality (Legler *et al.*, 1999). Linet *et al.* (1999) also report a relatively smaller reduction in childhood brain tumour mortality in the United States over the period 1975–1995 when compared to the reduction in leukaemia mortality and suggests that this represents the differing progress in developing effective therapies for these two diagnostic groups.

When we consider data from the NRCT series together with those from other available sources, it appears that the reductions in overall childhood cancer mortality in general and leukaemia mortality in particular up until the mid-1990s are somewhat smaller and occur later than those in the United States. This probably reflects the delay in implementing the most effective treatment regimes (Levi *et al.*, 2001) and indicates that further reductions in mortality are possible. Our data for the more recent years show that there has been a continuing reduction of 8.1% in overall cancer mortality (10.8% boys, 4.7% girls) and 11.4% in leukaemia mortality (13.4% boys, 8.8% girls) between 1995–1999 and 2000–2004, suggesting that reductions in mortality are still taking place. Mortality in children diagnosed with brain tumours has also decreased by 9.6% between 1995–1999 and 2000–2004, but the decrease in mortality was much more marked in boys (16.3%) than in girls (1.2%). Examination of the mortality data by age group shows that these recent decreases in mortality are almost entirely the result of marked reductions in infant cancer mortality.

6.3 The contribution of cancer to total childhood mortality

Deaths occurring in children diagnosed with a malignant neoplasm were also considered as a percentage of all deaths occurring for the same age group. Infants and children aged 1–14 were considered separately because general infant mortality patterns and rates are quite different from those of older children. In infants, cancer mortality as a percentage of total mortality was low throughout the study period: 0.33% in 1965–69, rising to 0.59% in 1995–1999 then falling sharply to 0.42% in 2000–2004 (Fig. 6.14). Cancer deaths represented a higher proportion of total deaths for infant girls than infant boys throughout the period, but by 2000–2004 the difference between the two sexes was very small.

In contrast, mortality among children aged 1–14 with cancer represents a significant proportion of the total mortality of that age group (Fig. 6.15). Deaths in children with cancer represented 15% of the total deaths in 1965–1969, and this had risen to 21% by 2000–2004; general child mortality fell faster over this period than childhood cancer mortality. Cancer mortality represented a slightly higher percentage of total mortality for girls than boys during the majority of the study period. Looking in more detail at the different age groups, since 1990–1994, there has been no difference between boys and girls aged 1–4 in the percentage of deaths accounted for by children with cancer (Fig. 6.16) and a very small difference in those aged 5–9 (Fig. 6.17). Mortality among girls with cancer aged 10–14

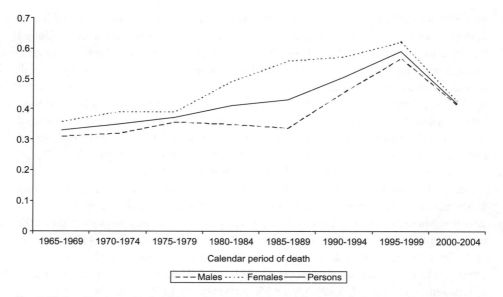

Fig. 6.14 Deaths at age 0 of children diagnosed with a malignant neoplasm as a percentage of all deaths for the same age group.

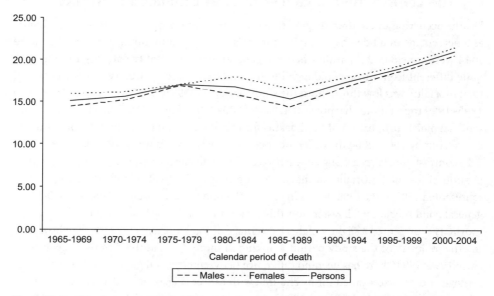

Fig. 6.15 Deaths at ages 1–14 of children diagnosed with a malignant neoplasm as a percentage of all deaths in the same age group.

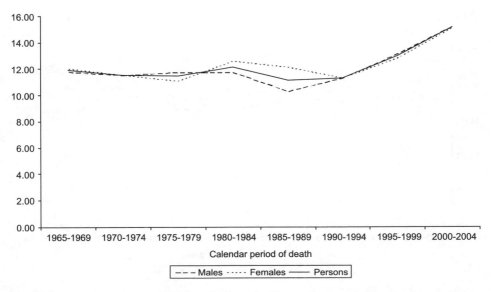

Fig. 6.16 Deaths at age 1–4 of children diagnosed with a malignant neoplasm as a percentage of all deaths in the same age group.

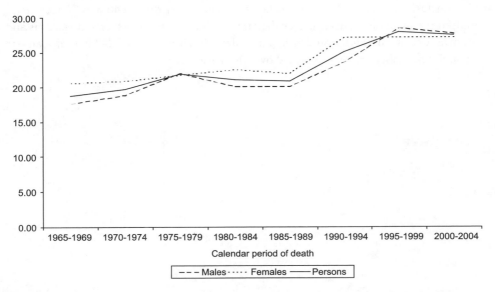

Fig. 6.17 Deaths at age 5–9 of children diagnosed with a malignant neoplasm as a percentage of all deaths in the same age group.

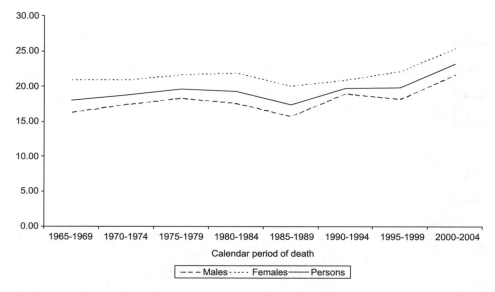

Fig. 6.18 Deaths at age 10–14 of children diagnosed with a malignant neoplasm as a percentage of all deaths in the same age group.

represented 21% of all cancer deaths in girls of that age in 1965–1969, compared to only 16% for boys. By 2000–2004, these figures had risen to 25 and 22%, respectively (Fig. 6.18).

In conclusion, childhood cancer mortality has fallen over the last 40 years, largely as a result of the increase in survival over the same period. Nevertheless, cancer remains an important cause of childhood death, particularly in children aged 1–14, as all-causes childhood mortality has also decreased over this period.

Chapter 7

Uses of the NRCT

MFG Murphy and AM Bayne

7.1 Background

The origins of the NRCT have been described in Chapter 1 and Chapter 2, as well as in related literature (Stiller *et al.*, 1995). The NRCT is committed to exploiting the multiple sources of data that contribute to its completeness, without compromising on the timeliness with which this can be achieved. Consequently, it is the most important supranational, population-based, specialist children's cancer registry in the world when considering its longevity, size of population at risk and depth and quality of information. Among its important constituent sources are the regional specialist children's tumour registries, namely the Northern Region Young Persons' (formerly Children's) Malignant Disease Registry, Manchester Children's Tumour Registry, West Midlands Regional Children's Tumour Registry, Yorkshire Specialist Register of Cancer in Children and Young People and the Bristol Childhood Cancer Research Registry. They offer comparable or even more detailed possibilities for data exploitation and rapid reporting of timely results (e.g. about time trends), but have the particular limitations of size (being local) and migration (relatively arbitrary, local boundaries). Nonetheless, without them the NRCT would be more limited in its functions. Much research of significance in its own right has been achieved within these local registries, and this can also serve to generate hypotheses for testing in the rest of the NRCT dataset. These registries are specialist for children, and some for young adults also, but cover all tumours in the age group. Several other specialist all-ages tumour registries have also helped the CCRG in its research and NRCT registration, most notably the leukaemia registries that collaborated in a study of adolescents and young adults (Stiller *et al.*, 1999; Benjamin *et al.*, 2000) and the bone tumour registries that assisted in a study of bone sarcoma diagnosed up to age 40 (Stiller *et al.*, 2006c).

Research is a principal function of the NRCT and of the CCRG, which houses it. However, the NRCT has a number of other uses in terms of audit and documentation of service provision. The dividing line between the two is unclear, so perhaps the best distinction is between descriptive and analytical studies that can be carried out using the routinely collected NRCT data and those that can only be accomplished by additional data collection based on NRCT records, whether by the CCRG or by others, e.g. the British Childhood Cancer Survivor Study (BCCSS), described later. The CCRG has access to non-NRCT datasets within the UK, such as the Oxford Record Linkage Study (Murphy *et al.*, 2001) and, internationally, e.g. the Utah Genealogy (Neale *et al.*, 2005), to accomplish other research objectives, but these are not considered here.

The bulk of the NRCT data are cancer registration records from regional and national (England and Wales, Scotland and Northern Ireland) all-ages cancer registries. These records are more basic than the relatively rich data collected at diagnosis by UK Children's Cancer Study Group (UKCCSG) clinicians for children under their care. Additional data, e.g. immunophenotype and treatment details, are collected at the time of entry into Childhood Leukaemia Working Party (CLWP) trials or during registration through UKCCSG. These two organizations merged in 2006 (see Chapter 2). The records of the specialist local children's registries are also rich but cover a much smaller proportion of patients. The NRCT receives all death registrations to age 20 years with cancer as the underlying cause but, in the few cases where registration is based on death certification only, there is little information apart from the cause of death. In addition, the CCRG is able to obtain the publicly available part of the birth registration details for over 90% of the children in the NRCT who were born in Britain; adoption is one of the main reasons for birth records being unavailable to us. This enhances the dataset available for assessing exposures around the time of the child's birth in relation to the initial tumour diagnosis, the second tumour in about 1% of cases and to survival and cause specific mortality.

A recurrent obligation before making any use of the data is to check their reliability and validity. Data obtained from the statutory civil registration systems for births and deaths are considered completely registered. More attention needs to be paid to whether the voluntary system of cancer registration maintains its effectiveness over time. The CCRG takes every opportunity to explore these issues using regular data exchanges, internal validation of the consistency of the data and checks with other independent data sources that might provide a comparator (Draper et al., 1991). These methods are fraught with assumptions, and we are occasionally notified of the small numbers of cases of which we were previously unaware. However, we believe the cancer registration process has been efficient and effective since the 1970s, and we are confident that few cancers were missed in the 1960s. We believe the registration data can be used to explore patterns of cancer incidence, survival, cause-specific mortality and second tumour occurrence from 1962 to the present day. In the cause of timeliness, we have settled on the compromise of declaring provisional completeness about 3 years in arrears. At the time of this writing, the NRCT is considered complete to 2002 inclusive, with 2003–04 in prospect.

7.2 Monitoring incidence, survival and mortality

The basic public health surveillance role and descriptive epidemiological research capacities of the NRCT merge into one another when categorising temporal and geographical variations in the occurrence of childhood tumours or survival after diagnosis. The smaller, regional childhood cancer registries and the NRCT interact, describing the patterns and interpreting the reasons for time trends evident in both local and national data (McNally et al., 1999, 2000; Feltbower et al., 2001; Kroll et al., 2006). The national picture for both haematological and solid malignancies is described extensively elsewhere in this book. Cause-specific mortality is not routinely analysed by the CCRG, though it may be in special circumstances (Robertson et al., 1992, 1994). This is in part due to the different methods used to derive and classify causes of death when using the totality of information available within the NRCT, compared to the tabulation of national mortality statistics by ONS and GRO(S) (Hawkins *et al.*, 1990; Campbell *et al.*, 2004). All-cause mortality data on fact and timing of death (and embarkation data) are used extensively in the detailed analysis of overall survival by specific tumour type and to eliminate deceased cohort members from the population at risk when studying the occurrence of second tumours.

The national data, usually for England and Wales only, have also contributed to international comparisons of incidence and survival trends and point estimates within Europe and around the world (Parkin *et al.*, 1988b, 1998; Gatta *et al.*, 2002). Within Europe, detailed analyses of incidence and survival have been coordinated as part of the EUROCARE (Capocaccia, Gatta, Magnani, Stiller, Coebergh, (Editors) 2001; Gatta *et al.*, 2003, 2005) and ACCIS (Automated Childhood Cancer Incidence System) projects (Steliarova-Foucher *et al.*, 2004, 2005a), shedding light on the comparative effectiveness of medical care systems organized in different ways and on possible aetiological factors. The Study for Evaluation of Neuroblastoma Screening in Europe (Powell *et al.*, 1998) evaluated neuroblastoma patterns in Austria, France, Germany and the UK, concluding that registration rates in infancy were related to different national patterns in child health examinations. The European Childhood Leukaemia/Lymphoma Incidence Study reported concerted European analysis of childhood leukaemia distributions after Chernobyl (Parkin *et al.*, 1993). In a series of papers based on registry data, the EUROCLUS study reported space–time clustering across Europe, which might suggest roles for a variety of environmental agents in causing childhood leukaemia (Alexander, 1998; Alexander *et al.*, 1998, 1999). Other even more specific comparisons between the UK trends and those in countries further afield are also possible and may be informative, e.g. neuroblastoma in Japan to assess the impact of screening (Honjo *et al.*, 2003), childhood melanoma in Australia to assess the impact of more intensely undertaken health protection measures or hepatic tumours in the Gambia to assess the impact of HBV vaccination. For some time-trend analyses, sophisticated statistical regression methods are needed based on time-series analyses. These allow for year-to-year correlation in both cancers observed and exposures assessed, e.g. the prevalence of specific infections as measured by the Health Protection Agency. Similar complicated modelling, such as age, period and cohort modelling, can be needed when assessing time-trends, the age distribution of cancers by single year of age, or both, as presented more simply elsewhere in this book (Draper *et al.*, 1994; Little *et al.*, 1996).

7.3 UKCCSG and Childhood Leukaemia Working Party Collaboration

The UKCCSG and CLWP clinical trial databases assist greatly in maintaining the completeness and depth of the NRCT's cancer registration process. The MRC Leukaemia Trials Office and, subsequently, the Clinical Trial Service Unit in Oxford have provided details of children entered to trials since the early 1970s. The UKCCSG has provided details of children under the care of its members since its inception in 1977 (UKCCSG, 2002).

The proportion of children registered on the NRCT who are first notified through a UKCCSG clinician has increased steadily and has now reached about 90%. This set of registrations of children (and young adults) is now the principal primary data source for the NRCT, though we may be notified of the same children with cancer from several sources. The CLWP trials database is another distinct source of data. The referral patterns for UKCCSG-registered patients and survival patterns for nearly every separable tumour type are calculated annually, spanning periods of the UKCCSG's existence since 1977 and reflecting the different eras in which children with relevant tumours were entered to successive clinical trials. These figures are published in the registry section of the UKCCSG annual report and on the membership section of the UKCCSG website.

Data for children registered by UKCCSG clinicians, or those entered to CLWP trials have been examined, with regard to factors that may be associated both with the likelihood of entry to a particular clinical trial and to clinical outcome of treatment. This has enabled the CCRG to investigate the effect on outcome of UKCCSG centre size, entry to trials and treatment on favoured protocols in operation at particular times. Detailed comparisons, 10 years apart, of the proportions of children with acute lymphoblastic leukaemia managed in specialist centres and the survival of these children have suggested the importance for the outcome of where patients are managed, entry to national clinical trials and increasing standardization of care within designated centres (Stiller and Draper, 1989; Stiller and Eatock, 1999). From these kinds of studies, quite strong evidence has emerged of the benefits of entry to trials, protocol-defined treatment and management by multidisciplinary specialist paediatric oncology teams (Lennox et al., 1979; Eden et al., 1988; Sanders et al., 1988; Stiller, 1988, 1994a).

Because UKCCSG clinicians have not always been responsible for registering the majority of certain kinds of childhood tumours, it is possible to compare outcomes including survival, second tumours and cause-specific mortality between children who were registered by UKCCSG clinicians and those who were not, while paying due attention to the age, sex and period of diagnosis. This also allows the possibility of assessing the likely effects of treatment-on-protocol adopted at the time, versus not, and possible effects of under/over treatment (Pritchard et al., 1989).

Reconciliation of the NRCT data with those available when children are entered to UKCCSG or CLWP trials also results in the validation or correction of the principal tumour diagnosis and the collection of more detailed data on pathology (e.g. immunophenotypes) and treatment than the NRCT might collect at the time of initial registration.

Another benefit of the professional centralization that the existence of the NRCT allied to the UKCCSG and CLWP networks offers is an ability to maintain an interest, from both aetiological and treatment points of view, in paediatric tumours that are truly rare, and encountered by few. The NRCT is able to provide population-based information about rare tumours and also some borderline malignancies such as myelodysplasia for which it holds and maintains a national register (Kardos et al., 2003; Passmore et al., 2003). Synthesis of clinical observations and the simple epidemiology (who, what, when, where) of these conditions allows a coherent description of the state of knowledge of tumours of which few will have first-hand experience (Walker et al., 2002; Brennan et al., 2004).

7.4 Geographical epidemiology

There is little universal agreement about the nature and strength of associations of different tumour types with population characteristics, partly because childhood cancers are comparatively rare and difficult to study in detail on a large scale. Simple descriptions of temporal, social and geographical variations in the occurrence of childhood tumours in large populations still have a distinct place in defining what can be said to be known about the childhood cancers. To study potential causes, the NRCT data resource can be analysed in relation to demographic and environmental data available for geographical areas of Britain and in relation to specific locations of exposures that may be harmful.

These investigations may be conducted by simply using data available on the place of birth and diagnosis or, for place-of-birth analyses, by using the population-based set of birth registration control data (described below) available for each case together with its own birth registration details. Information about exposure to ionising radiation as judged by maps of exposure to radon (daughters) and gamma radiation has been used to assess risks of childhood leukaemia (Richardson *et al.*, 1995). Future analyses might, e.g., include assessing latitude-based measures of UV exposure for childhood melanoma or retinoblastoma (Jemal *et al.*, 2000). Similarly, the relationship between the fluoride content of water supplies and risk of bone tumours (in particular) could also be assessed (Bassin *et al.*, 2006; Douglass and Joshipura, 2006), as could any other environmental exposure that is broadly mappable to administrative areas or specific postcode aggregations.

Much more detailed assessment of likely exposure may sometimes be made based on physical distances from sources of exposure. A good example of this is the work on potential exposure to electromagnetic fields (EMF), as measured by distance from power lines, and childhood leukaemia (Draper *et al.*, 2005). Others have used data similar to those held by the NRCT to calculate risks from exposure to products of internal combustion engines (Knox, 2005a,,b, 2006). Similarly, great use has been made of NRCT data, particularly in an extensive series of reports by the Committee on Medical Aspects of Radiation in the Environment (COMARE), to assess the importance of residence in the vicinity of a variety of nuclear installations in relation to childhood cancer occurrence (Bithell *et al.*, 1994; Committee on Medical Aspects of Radiation in the Environment (COMARE), 2005). Its most recent report (COMARE, 2006) includes other types of related geographical analyses that the data make possible, e.g. assessments of any general tendencies of the different kinds of childhood tumours to cluster in space, and of tendencies to exhibit space–time clustering (McNally *et al.*, 2006). Additionally, this report employs analyses involving regressions of childhood cancer occurrence in small administrative areas on 'ecological' features of those areas, such as census-based measures of socioeconomic status, overcrowding, urban/rural status, and population density. Particular attention has also been paid to analyses based on measures of population mixing to shed light on infection-related hypotheses of childhood leukaemia occurrence (Kinlen *et al.*, 1991, 1995; Stiller and Boyle, 1996).

One final example of uses to which NRCT data are put in terms of geographical analysis is that of assisting in public health investigation and evaluation of the significance of cancer clusters that come to public attention, and in the investigation of acute environmental contamination incidents (Lyons *et al.*, 1995; Bithell and Draper, 1999; Owen *et al.*, 2002).

7.5 **The NRCT as a source of case (and control) data**

The NRCT holds relatively rich datasets when compared to the nonspecialist registries. These data are used in their own right or in conjunction with other information collected by the CCRG. They may also be used as the basis of studies carried out by researchers outside the CCRG, often with CCRG involvement.

As a cancer registry, the NRCT is currently covered by the exemption granted to the UK Association of Cancer Registries by the Patient Information Advisory Group (PIAG), under Section 60 of the Health and Social Care Act (2001), from the need to obtain individual consent for its data holdings or to undertake anonymization of its data. The NRCT contains the permitted identifying information about each child at the time of diagnosis together with, in most instances, the publicly available details from the child's birth registration document. This information makes studies of the extent to which siblings are affected with childhood cancers a great deal easier (Draper *et al.*, 1977, 1992, 1996). For each set of birth registration details, a control set of birth registration details for an unaffected child are also held. The control child is of the same sex, born around the same time and living in the same local area at the time of birth as the case child. These data were assembled for specific record linkage studies but create the opportunity for a number of other uses (Draper *et al.*, 1997a,b; Sorahan *et al.*, 2003).

Registrations received from UKCCSG clinicians include a limited amount of additional data, e.g. a statement of ethnicity and the presence of congenital malformations detected in the child. It is then possible to compile subsets of cases for further more detailed studies such as children with cancer and a history of neurofibromatosis (Stiller *et al.*, 1994) or children affected by both leukaemia and Down, or other, syndromes (Robertson and Hawkins, 1995; Narod *et al.*, 1997; Satgé *et al.*, 1998; Rao *et al.*, 2006). Having obtained all the relevant permissions, the NRCT has recently identified the small number of children with tumours and overgrowth syndromes for a study of the genetic basis of such co-occurrence. Use of ethnicity data notified by UKCCSG clinicians also allows some further analyses of variations in childhood cancer occurrence (Stiller *et al.*, 1991a) and survival (Stiller *et al.*, 2000).

As mentioned previously, the birth record data for cases and controls may be the essential basis of a study. The study of EMF described in the earlier section on geographical epidemiology was based on knowledge of the physical distance from the address at birth of the cases and controls to the power lines that were the object of the investigation. When the issue of routine vitamin K administration and subsequent childhood cancer risk was being investigated, the NRCT birth data were used to locate the hospital maternity units in question, and studies of two different designs were used. One was a case-control study, comparing the records of vitamin K administration between childhood cancer cases and controls selected from the same hospital's birth registers, rather than the standard CCRG controls. The other compared the rates of childhood cancer occurrence among children born in particular hospitals with different "average" vitamin K policies, compared to the number that would have been expected based on the total number of children born there in a defined period (Passmore *et al.*, 1998a,b).

In a limited way, the information contained in the publicly available birth registration details of cases and controls can itself be informative about exposures of interest without much further data gathering. A statement of the father's occupation, and much less frequently the mother's, is made at birth registration and recorded there, allowing studies of occupational associations with case/control status to be undertaken. Birth registration details can also be used to explore issues such as whether being a member of a multiple birth has any effect on cancer risk and twin concordance for cancer (Buckley *et al.*, 1996; Murphy *et al.*, 2001). With special precautions employed along with additional permissions, such data have also been used to assess the effect of mother's age and parity (Dockerty *et al.*, 2001), and will be used to assess birthweight-related effects in cases and controls in the future.

As discussed in Chapter 2 and Chapter 5, the NRCT is able to identify subsequent primary tumours developing in surviving children who have been traced and flagged at NHSCR, so long as they stay in Britain, because the (all-ages) cancer registries themselves notify all their registrations to NHSCR (Draper *et al.*, 1986; Hawkins *et al.*, 1987, 1992; Kingston *et al.*, 1987; Hawkins, 1989; Hawkins and Swerdlow, 1992; Menu-Branthomme *et al.*, 2004; Jenkinson *et al.*, 2004). Why subsequent primary tumours occur is of great interest, and study of their relation to treatments used for the first tumour can be undertaken, with appropriate permissions obtained to allow retrieval of data from the case notes. Data on children surviving 5 years from their diagnosis have been used to generate population-based long-term follow-up studies (Hawkins *et al.*, 1988; Hawkins and Smith, 1989). These include the British Childhood Cancer Survivor Study (BCCSS), now based in Birmingham, which involves the collection of large amounts of information from each survivor by postal questionnaire about many aspects of their lives since the original diagnosis and covering the full range of childhood tumours (Taylor *et al.*, 2004).

Even more sophisticated future studies might be conducted with suitable permissions in the future. Since the late 1970s in England and Wales, and earlier in Scotland, Guthrie blood spots (the heel pinprick specimens used to screen for inborn errors of metabolism, particularly phenylketonuria) have been retained by some regional screening programmes, and some remain retrievable based on a knowledge of where a childhood cancer case or control was born. The CCRG is exploring the possibility of examining these tissue specimens for genetic and other characteristics that might be related to risk. Similarly, where the molecular characteristics of the mutation in hereditary retinoblastoma cases are known, they might be used to study the impact of the type of mutation on the subsequent course of the disease.

7.6 Individual record linkage studies

The identifying information held for cases in the NRCT, together with the matched set of birth controls, can be used, with permissions, to link to other data held about these individuals.

As described above, the cancer registries including the NRCT use standard tracing and flagging mechanisms to determine the occurrence of subsequent primary tumours and the detail of deaths that occur, in order to study survival and cause of death. Occasionally, it is possible to study other outcomes by record linkage, and jointly the UKCCSG and CCRG have PIAG permission for an updated study involving individual record linkage to UK Transplant. The study will look at the extent of cardiac transplantation in childhood cancer survivors and also the relationship between the chemotherapy used to treat the child's original tumour and the need for this surgery (Levitt et al., 1996).

More frequently, record linkage is used to relate the fact of occurrence of the first childhood cancer to the details of exposure at an individual level, in a group exposed in this way. Good identifiers on both the exposure records and the NRCT are needed for this to be successful. The possible lack of such identifiers, as well as legal reasons, prevented the CCRG from pursuing linkage of Human Fertilisation and Embryology Authority records to those of the NRCT, in order to further study the childhood cancer risk in babies conceived following in vitro fertilization and other assisted reproduction technology procedures after the initial cohort report (Doyle et al., 1998). However, good identifying details exist for at least one other UK cohort of women successfully treated for subfertility;therefore, the study of cancer risk in children born to women who experienced subfertility treatments remains a possibility worth pursuing (Lightfoot et al., 2005).

Other examples of record linkage studies, for which a variety of permissions is always sought before proceeding, include a linkage of the birth registration data for all cases and controls to the records of men and women who might have become parents while working in jobs that involved exposure to ionising radiation, thus enabling the study of cancer risk in their children (Draper et al., 1997a,b; Sorahan et al., 2003). Related and more complicated parent/child designs can also be pursued by different means. Examples include determining cancer status in women who gave birth to twins before linkage of the twin baby cohort records to those of the NRCT in order to study familial clustering of cancer risk, or accomplishing the same for the cohort of women mentioned above who delivered after experiencing a period of subfertility. Simpler examples include the renewed interest in the occurrence of childhood cancer in babies born to a cohort of women who underwent radiological pelvimetric assessment during pregnancy in the 1940s and 1950s (Court Brown et al., 1960), and an intended study of the risk of childhood tumours in children who underwent computerized tomographic (CT) scanning for a variety of reasons.

In the future, increased use of NHS numbers will make possible a variety of linkage studies involving the NRCT, including those of potentially greater interest in terms of health services usage rather than to shed light on aetiology. For instance, it is becoming possible to identify admissions of children with cancer in the Hospital Episode Statistics (HES) and Cancer Waiting Times (CWT) statistical systems, and to link their records to provide a narrative account of hospitalization before and after the cancer diagnosis admission. This may be extended to include radiotherapy, outpatient and day case records, and this may allow the further collection and analysis of data on treatment and treatment-related complications, as well as providing a confirmatory check on data items that the NRCT obtains by other means, e.g. statements of ethnicity. Although they would not need to involve linkage to the NRCT, studies using general practice databases of exposure and patterns of consulting prior to the diagnosis of childhood cancer may also be possible and useful.

7.7 Other functions of the registry

The constant attention to Registry activities means the ready availability of a certain, limited dataset on a large population of individuals with childhood cancer. Coding and classification expertise has been developed through constant practice, and the NRCT acts as a source of specific advice on this and other more general matters to others working in the field (Steliarova-Foucher *et al.*, 2005b).

It is also a general information resource, providing a wide range of basic information and childhood cancer statistics in the UK (Kroll *et al.*, 2004) and answering queries from members of the public and charities with an interest in many issues relating to childhood cancer. Since 2005, basic data from the NRCT, in the form of incidence and survival rates, have been presented and are downloadable from the CCRG website http://www.ccrg.ox.ac.uk. These data are updated as each new diagnosis year is declared complete. Individuals and organizations requiring access to the data for a variety of purposes need to be instructed in the necessary levels of permissions that must be obtained, such as from the UKCCSG Epidemiology and Registries Group, Multi Centre Research Ethics Committee or PIAG when the request cannot be simply met, and how to obtain these permissions expeditiously. Data are distributed to outside users at the rate of about one request per week, and enquiries to the Registry about childhood cancer matters occur with the same frequency.

With suitable agreements in place, large datasets can be distributed and used in the development of new methods to analyse childhood cancer occurrence and survival, and can form the basis of higher university degree studies (Shah, 2005).

7.8 The future

It is unlikely that the NRCT will directly collect ever larger amounts of data in the future about children with cancer. Issues of practicality and data protection make this difficult to do well. As suggested above, however, an increase in pseudonymized record linkage using unique NHS numbers to datasets held within the NHS and elsewhere is likely to be the basis for enriching the range of studies that the NRCT makes possible. These data will probably relate to exposure of both the child and parents at potentially sensitive times, to study aetiology, and to the consequences of having childhood cancer with regard to both treatment and healthcare. As relevant genetic data are accumulated (e.g. the nature of mutations in children with the heritable form of retinoblastoma), they too can be included and used to continue and enhance in new ways the population-based research, which has always been at the heart of the NRCT's work.

Concern about the effective, appropriate treatment of teenagers and young adults with cancer (Stevens, 2006), whose needs are significantly different from those of children, may mean that systematic registry-like information will need to be developed on a national scale for this age group as already happens in certain regions (Wilkinson *et al.*, 2001;

Pearce *et al.*, 2005). However, this may well not occur through a simple extension of the NRCT, although the bone sarcoma study undertaken by CCRG showed that it was possible to do this to an age of 40 years, but may be based on different methods of data accumulation.

The NRCT remains an exemplar of children's cancer registration, and advice sought from the NRCT has contributed to the thinking behind recent developments in childhood cancer registration in various countries around the world, notably Switzerland, India and the USA. The value of the special effort needed to achieve timely, complete childhood cancer registration is recognized, and we believe it has an important future.

References

Ablett S, Pinkerton CR, on behalf of the United Kingdom Children's Cancer Study Group (UKCCSG) (2003). Recruiting children into cancer trials – role of the United Kingdom Children's Cancer Study Group (UKCCSG). *British Journal of Cancer*, **88**, 1661–5.

Ajiki W, Tsukuma H, Oshima A, Kawa K (1998). Effects of mass screening for neuroblastoma on incidence, mortality, and survival rates in Osaka, Japan. *Cancer Causes & Control: CCC*, **9**, 631–6.

Ajiki W, Tsukuma H, Oshima A (2004). Survival rates of childhood cancer patients in Osaka, Japan. *Japanese Journal of Clinical Oncology*, **34**, 50–4.

Alexander F (1998). Clustering of childhood acute leukaemia. The EUROCLUS project. *Radiation and Environmental Biophysics*, **37**, 71–4.

Alexander FE, Boyle P, Carli PM *et al.* (1998). Spatial clustering of childhood leukaemia: summary results from the EUROCLUS project. *British Journal of Cancer*, **77**, 818–24.

Alexander FE, Boyle P, Carli PM *et al.* (1999). Population density and childhood leukaemia: Results of the EUROCLUS study. *European Journal of Cancer*, **35**, 439–44.

American Cancer Society. (1968). *Manual of Tumor Nomenclature and Coding*, 1968. American Cancer Society, Inc., Washington, DC.

Antonelli A, Miccoli P, Derzhitski VE, Panasiuk G, Solovieva N, Baschieri L (1996). Epidemiologic and clinical evaluation of thyroid cancer in children from the Gomel region (Belarus). *World Journal of Surgery*, **20**, 867–71.

Asmar L, Gehan EA, Newton WA *et al.* (1994). Agreement among and within groups of pathologists in the classification of rhabdomyosarcoma and related childhood sarcomas: Report of an International study of four pathology classifications. *Cancer*, **74**, 2579–88.

Atra A, Gerrard M, Hobson R *et al.* (1998). Improved cure rate in children with B-cell acute lymphoblastic leukaemia (B-ALL) and stage IV B-cell non-Hodgkin's lymphoma (B-NHL) – results of the UKCCSG 9003 protocol. *British Journal of Cancer*, **77**, 2281–5.

Atra A, Higgs E, Capra M *et al.* (2002). ChIVPP chemotherapy in children with stage IV Hodgkin's disease: results of the UKCCSG HD 8201 and HD 9201 studies. *British Journal of Haematology*, **119**, 647–51.

Atra A, Imeson JD, Hobson R *et al.* (2000). Improved outcome in children with advanced-stage B-cell non-Hodgkin's lymphoma (B-NHL): results of the United Kingdom Children's Cancer Study Group (UKCCSG) 9002 protocol. *British Journal of Cancer*, **82**, 1396–402.

Bailey CC, Gnekow A, Wellek S *et al.* (1995). Prospective randomised trial of chemotherapy given before radiotherapy in childhood medulloblastoma. International Society of Paediatric Oncology (SIOP) and the (German) Society of Paediatric Oncology (GPO): SIOP II. *Medical and Pediatric Oncology*, **25**, 166–78.

Barnes E (2005). Caring and curing: paediatric cancer services since 1960. *European Journal of Cancer Care*, **14**, 373–80.

Bassin EB, Wypij D, Davis RB, Mittleman MA (2006). Age-specific fluoride exposure in drinking water and osteosarcoma (United States). *Cancer Causes & Control: CCC*, **17**, 421–8.

Becroft DMO, Dockerty JD, Berkeley BB *et al.* (1999). Childhood cancer in New Zealand 1990 to 1993. *Pathology*, **31**, 83–9.

Benjamin S, Kroll ME, Cartwright RA *et al.* (2000). Haematologists' approaches to the management of adolescents and young adults with acute leukaemia. *British Journal of Haematology*, **111**, 1045–50.

Bernstein L, Gurney JG (1999). Carcinomas and other malignant epithelial neoplasms. In: Gloeckler Ries LA, Smith MA, Gurney JG, Linet M, Tamra T, Young JL, Bunin GR (eds.) *Cancer Incidence and*

Survival among Children and Adolescents: United States SEER Program 1975–1995, NIH Pub No 99–4649, Bethesda, MD, pp. 139–47.

Bernstein L, Linet M, Smith MA, Olshan AF (1999a). Renal tumors. In: Gloeckler Ries LA, Smith MA, Gurney JG, Linet M, Tamra T, Young JL, Bunin GR (eds.) *Cancer Incidence and Survival among Children and Adolescents: United States SEER Program 1975–1995*, NIH Pub No 99–4649, Bethesda, MD, pp. 79–90.

Bernstein L, Smith MA, Liu L, Deapen D, Friedman DL (1999b). Germ cell, trophoblastic and other gonadal neoplasms. In: Gloeckler Ries LA, Smith MA, Gurney JG, Linet M, Tamra T, Young JL, Bunin GR (eds.) *Cancer Incidence and Survival among Children and Adolescents: United States SEER Program 1975–1995*, NIH Pub No 99–4649, Bethesda, pp. MD, pp. 125–37.

Bernstein ML, Leclerc JM, Bunin G *et al.* (1992). A population-based study of neuroblastoma incidence, survival, and mortality in North America. *Journal of Clinical Oncology*, **10**, 323–9.

Biondi A, Cimino G, Pieters R, Pui C-H (2000). Biological and therapeutic aspects of infant leukemia. *Blood*, **96**, 24–33.

Birch JM (1988). United Kingdom – Manchester Children's Tumour Registry 1954–1970 and 1971–1983. In: Parkin DM *et al.* (eds.) *International Incidence of Childhood Cancer*, IARC, Lyon, pp. 299–304.

Birch JM, Marsden HB (1987). A classification scheme for childhood cancer. *International Journal of Cancer*, **40**, 620–4.

Bithell JF, Draper GJ (1999). Uranium-235 and childhood leukaemia around Greenham Common airfield. *Journal of Radiological Protection*, **19**, 253–9.

Bithell JF, Dutton SJ, Draper GJ, Neary NM (1994). The distribution of childhood leukaemias and non-Hodgkin lymphomas near nuclear installations in England and Wales. *British Medical Journal*, **309**, 501–5.

Black WC (1998). Increasing incidence of childhood primary malignant brain tumors – enigma or no-brainer? *Journal of the National Cancer Institute*, **90**, 1249–51.

Boque A, Wilson RG (1977). Chronic myeloid leukaemia of adult type in 5-month-old infant. *Br Med J*, **2**, 1397.

Bramwell VHC, Burgers M, Sneath R *et al.* (1992). A comparison of two short intensive adjuvant chemotherapy regimens in operable osteosarcoma of limbs in children and young adults: The first study of the European Osteosarcoma Intergroup. *Journal of Clinical Oncology*, **10**, 1579–91.

Brennan BMD, Foot ABM, Stiller C *et al.* (2004). Where to next with extracranial rhabdoid tumours in children. *European Journal of Cancer*, **40**, 624–6.

Breslow N, Beckwith JB, Ciol M, Sharples K (1988). Age distribution of Wilms' tumor: report from the National Wilms' Tumor Study. *Cancer Research*, **48**, 1653–7.

Breslow N, McCann B (1971). Statistical estimation of prognosis for children with neuroblastoma. *Cancer Research*, **31**, 2098–103.

Buckley JD, Buckley CM, Breslow NE, Draper GJ, Roberson PK, Mack TM (1996). Concordance for childhood cancer in twins. *Medical and Pediatric Oncology*, **26**, 223–9.

Bulterys M, Goodman MT, Smith MA, Buckley JD (1999). Hepatic tumors. In: Gloeckler Ries LA, Smith MA, Gurney JG, Linet M, Tamra T, Young JL, Bunin GR (eds.) *Cancer Incidence and Survival among Children and Adolescents: United States SEER Program 1975–1995*, NIH Pub No 99–4649, Bethesda, MD, pp. 91–7.

Bunin GR, Surawicz TS, Witman PA, Preston-Martin S, Davis F, Bruner JM (1998). The descriptive epidemiology of craniopharyngioma. *Journal of Neurosurgery*, **89**, 547–51.

Burke GAA, Imeson J, Hobson R, Gerrard M (2003). Localized non-Hodgkin's lymphoma with B-cell histology: cure without cyclophosphamide? A report of the United Kingdom Children's Cancer Study Group on studies NHL 8501 and NHL 9001 (1985–1996). *British Journal of Haematology*, **121**, 586–91.

Burkhardt B, Zimmermann M, Oschlies I *et al.* (2005). The impact of age and gender on biology, clinical features and treatment outcome of non-Hodgkin lymphoma in childhood and adolescence. *British Journal of Haematology*, **131**, 39–49.

Campbell J, Wallace WHB, Bhatti LA, Stockton DL, Rapson T, Brewster DH (eds.) (2004). *Childhood Cancer in Scotland: trends in incidence, mortality, and survival 1975–1999*. Information & Statistics Division, Edinburgh.

Capocaccia R, Gatta G, Magnani C, Stiller C, Coebergh J-W, (eds.) (2001). Childhood cancer survival in Europe 1978–1992: the EUROCARE study (special issue). *European Journal of Cancer*, **37**, 671–816.

Carli M, Colombatti R, Oberlin O *et al.* (2004). European intergroup studies (MMT4-89 and MMT4-91) on childhood metastatic rhabdomyosarcoma: final results and analysis of prognostic factors. *Journal of Clinical Oncology*, **22**, 4787–94.

Cartwright RA, Gurney KA, Moorman AV (2002). Sex ratios and the risks of haematological malignancies. *British Journal of Haematology*, **118**, 1071–7.

CBTRUS (2002). Statistical report: Primary brain tumors in the United States, 1995–1999. Central Brain Tumor Registry of the United States.

Chang M-H, Chen C-J, Lai M-S *et al.* (1997). Universal hepatitis B vaccination in Taiwan and the incidence of hepatocellular carcinoma in children. *New England Journal of Medicine*, **336**, 1855–9.

Chessells JM (1992). Chronic myeloid leukaemia, myeloproliferative disorders, and myelodysplasia. In: Lilleyman JS, Hann IM (eds.) *Paediatric Haematology*, Churchill Livingstone, pp. 59–63.

Chessells JM, Eden OB, Bailey CC, Lilleyman JS, Richards SM (1994). Acute lymphoblastic leukaemia in infancy: experience in MRC UKALL trials. Report from the Medical Research Council Working Party on Childhood Leukaemia. *Leukemia*, **8**, 1275–9.

Chessells JM, Harrison CJ, Kempski H *et al.* (2002a). Clinical features, cytogenetics and outcome in acute lymphoblastic and myeloid leukaemia of infancy: report from the MRC Childhood Leukaemia working party. *Leukemia*, **16**, 776–84.

Chessells JM, Harrison CJ, Watson SL, Vora AJ, Richards SM (2002b). Treatment of infants with lymphoblastic leukaemia: results of the UK infant protocols 1987–1999. *British Journal of Haematology*, **117**, 306–14.

Chessells JM, Harrison G, Richards SM *et al.* (2002c). Failure of a new protocol to improve treatment results in paediatric lymphoblastic leukaemia: lessons from the UK Medical Research Council trials UKALL X and UKALL XI. *British Journal of Haematology*, **118**, 445–55.

Chessells JM, Sieff CA, Rankin A (1983). Acute myeloid leukaemia in childhood: treatment in the United Kingdom. *Haematology and Blood Transfusion*, **28**, 51–5.

Clavel J, Goubin A, Auclerc MF *et al.* (2004). Incidence of childhood leukaemia and non-Hodgkin's lymphoma in France: National Registry of Childhood Leukaemia and Lymphoma, 1990–1999. *European Journal of Cancer Prevention*, **13**, 97–103.

Clavel J, Steliarova-Foucher E, Berger C, Danon S, Valerianova Z (2006). Hodgkin's disease incidence and survival in European children and adolescents (1978–1997): report from the ACCIS project. *European Journal of Cancer*, **42**, 2037–49.

Coebergh J-W, Reedijk AMJ, de Vries E *et al.* (2006). Leukaemia incidence and survival in children and adolescents in Europe during 1978–1997: report from the ACCIS project. *European Journal of Cancer*, **42**, 2019–36.

Cohn SL (1999). Diagnosis and classification of the small round-cell tumors of childhood. *Am J Pathol*, **155**, 11–5.

Committee on Medical Aspects of Radiation in the Environment (COMARE) (2005). COMARE 10th report: the incidence of childhood cancer around nuclear installations in Great Britain. Chilton, Didcot, Health Protection Agency.

Committee on Medical Aspects of Radiation in the Environment (COMARE) (2006). COMARE 11th report: The distribution of childhood leukaemia and other childhood cancer in Great Britain. Chilton, Didcot, Health Protection Agency.

Conter V, Aricò M, Valsecchi MG *et al.* (2000). Long-term results of the Italian Association of Pediatric Hematology and Oncology (AIEOP) acute lymphoblastic leukemia studies, 1982–1995. *Leukemia*, **14**, 2196–204.

Conti EMS, Cercato MC, Gatta G, Ramazzotti V, Roscioni S (2001). Childhood melanoma in Europe since 1978: a population-based survival study. *European Journal of Cancer*, **37**, 780–4.

Correa P and Chen VW (1995). Endocrine gland cancer. *Cancer*, **75**, 338–52.

Cotterill SJ, Ahrens S, Paulussen M *et al.* (2000a). Prognostic factors in Ewing's tumor of bone: analysis of 975 patients from the European Intergroup Cooperative Ewing's Sarcoma Study Group. *Journal of Clinical Oncology*, **18**, 3108–14.

Cotterill SJ, Parker L, Malcolm AJ, Reid M, More L, Craft AW (2000b). Incidence and survival for cancer in children and young adults in the north of England, 1968–1995: a report from the Northern Region Young Persons' Malignant Disease Registry. *British Journal of Cancer*, **83**, 397–403.

Cotterill SJ, Pearson ADJ, Pritchard J *et al.* (2000c). Clinical prognostic factors in 1277 patients with neuroblastoma: results of the European Neuroblastoma Study Group 'survey' 1982–1992. *European Journal of Cancer*, **36**, 901–8.

Court Brown WM, Doll R, Bradford Hill A (1960). Incidence of leukaemia after exposure to diagnostic radiation in utero. *British Medical Journal*, **5212**, 1539–45.

Craft A, Cotterill S, Malcolm A *et al.* (1998). Ifosfamide-containing chemotherapy in Ewing's sarcoma: The second United Kingdom Children's Cancer Study Group and the Medical Research Council Ewing's tumor study. *Journal of Clinical Oncology*, **16**, 3628–33.

Darbari A, Sabin KM, Shapiro CN, Schwarz KB (2003). Epidemiology of primary hepatic malignancies in U.S. children. *Hepatology*, **38**, 560–6.

Daugaard S (2004). Current soft-tissue sarcoma classifications. *European Journal of Cancer*, **40**, 543–8.

de Vries E, Steliarova-Foucher E, Spatz A, Eggermont AMM, Coebergh JWW (2006). Skin cancer incidence and survival in European children and adolescents (1978–1997): report from the ACCIS project. *European Journal of Cancer*, **42**, 2170–82.

Desandes E, Clavel J, Berger C *et al.* (2004). Cancer incidence among children in France, 1990–1999. *Pediatric Blood & Cancer*, **43**, 749–57.

Dockerty JD, Becroft DMO, Lewis ME, Williams SM (1997). The accuracy and completeness of childhood cancer registration in New Zealand. *Cancer Causes & Control: CCC*, **8**, 857–64.

Dockerty JD, Draper GJ, Vincent TJ, Rowan SD, Bunch KJ (2001). Case-control study of parental age, parity and socioeconomic level in relation to childhood cancers. *International Journal of Epidemiology*, **30**, 1428–37.

dos Santos Silva I, Swerdlow AJ (1993). Sex differences in the risks of hormone-dependent cancers. *American Journal of Epidemiology*, **138**, 10–28.

dos Santos Silva I, Swerdlow AJ, Stiller CA, Reid A (1999). Incidence of testicular germ-cell malignancies in England and Wales: trends in children compared with adults. *International Journal of Cancer*, **83**, 630–4.

Douglas NM, Dockerty JD (2005). Population-based survival of children in New Zealand diagnosed with cancer during 1990–1993. *European Journal of Cancer*, **41**, 1604–9.

Douglass CW, Joshipura K (2006). Caution needed in fluoride and osteosarcoma study. *Cancer Causes & Control: CCC*, **17**, 481–2.

Doyle P, Bunch KJ, Beral V, Draper GJ (1998). Cancer incidence in children conceived with assisted reproduction technology (research letter). *Lancet*, **352**, 452–3.

Draper G, Vincent T, Kroll ME, Swanson J (2005). Childhood cancer in relation to distance from high-voltage power lines in England and Wales: a case-control study. *British Medical Journal*, **330**, 1290–4.

Draper GJ, Birch JM, Bithell JF *et al.* (1982). Childhood cancer in Britain: Incidence, mortality and survival, OPCS Studies on Medical and Population Subjects No. 37, HMSO, London.

Draper GJ, Heaf MM, Kinnier Wilson LM (1977). Occurrence of childhood cancers among sibs and estimation of familial risks. *Journal of Medical Genetics*, **14**, 81–90.

Draper GJ, Kroll ME, Stiller CA (1994). Childhood Cancer. *Cancer Surveys*, **19/20**, 493–517.

Draper GJ, Little MP, Sorahan T *et al.* (1997a). Cancer in the offspring of radiation workers: a record linkage study. *British Medical Journal*, **315**, 1181–8.

Draper GJ, Little MP, Sorahan T *et al.* (1997b). *Cancer in the Offspring of Radiation Workers – a Record Linkage Study*, NRPB-R298. NRPB, Didcot.

Draper GJ, Sanders BM, Brownbill PA, Hawkins MM (1992). Patterns of risk of hereditary retinoblastoma and applications to genetic counselling. *British Journal of Cancer*, **66**, 211–9.

Draper GJ, Sanders BM, Kingston JE (1986). Second primary neoplasms in patients with retinoblastoma. *British Journal of Cancer*, **53**, 661–71.

Draper GJ, Sanders BM, Lennox EL, Brownbill PA (1996). Patterns of childhood cancer among siblings. *British Journal of Cancer*, **74**, 152–8.

Draper GJ, Stiller CA, O'Connor CM *et al.* (1991). Draper GJ (ed.) The Geographical Epidemiology of Childhood Leukaemia and Non-Hodgkin Lymphomas in Great Britain, 1966–83, OPCS Studies on Medical and Population Subjects No. 53, OPCS, London.

Dreifaldt AC, Carlberg M, Hardell L (2004). Increasing incidence rates of childhood malignant diseases in Sweden during the period 1960–1998. *European Journal of Cancer*, **40**, 1351–60.

Eden OB, Hann I, Imeson J, Cotterill S, Gerrard M, Pinkerton CR (1992). Treatment of advanced stage T cell lymphoblastic lymphoma: results of the United Kingdom Children's Cancer Study Group (UKCCSG) protocol 8503. *British Journal of Haematology*, **82**, 310–6.

Eden OB, Harrison G, Richards S *et al.* (2000). Long-term follow-up of the United Kingdom Medical Research Council protocols for childhood acute lymphoblastic leukaemia, 1980–1997. *Leukemia*, **14**, 2307–20.

Eden OB, Lilleyman JS, Richards S, Shaw MP, Peto J (1991). Results of Medical Research Council Childhood Leukaemia Trial UKALL VIII (Report to the Medical Research Council on behalf of the Working Party on Leukaemia in Childhood). *British Journal of Haematology*, **78**, 187–96.

Eden OB, Stiller CA, Gerrard MP (1988). Improved survival for childhood acute lymphoblastic leukemia: possible effect of protocol compliance. *Pediatric Hematology and Oncology*, **5**, 83–91.

Feltbower RG, Moorman AV, Dovey G, Kinsey SE, McKinney PA (2001). Incidence of childhood acute lymphoblastic leukaemia in Yorkshire, UK (research letter). *Lancet*, **358**, 385–7.

Ferlay J, Bray F, Pisani P, Parkin DM (2004). *GLOBOCAN 2002: Cancer Incidence, Mortality and Prevalence Worldwide*, IARC Cancerbase No. 5, version 2.0. IARC Press, Lyon.

Fine SW, Humphrey PA, Dehner LP, Amin MB, Epstein JI (2005). Urothelial neoplasms in patients 20 years or younger: a clinicopathological analysis using the World Health Organization 2004 bladder consensus classification. *The Journal of Urology*, **174**, 1976–80.

Foreman NK, Thorne R, Berry PJ, Oakhill A, Mott MG (1994). Childhood malignancies in the south-west region of England, 1976–1985. *Medical and Pediatric Oncology*, **23**, 14–9.

Gadner H, Grois N, Aricó M *et al.* (2001). A randomized trial of treatment for multisystem Langerhans' cell histiocytosis. *Journal of Pediatrics*, **138**, 728–34.

Gardiner CM, Reen DJ, O'Meara A (1995). Recognition of unusual presentation of natural killer cell leukemia. *American Journal of Hematology*, **50**, 133–9.

Gatta G, Capocaccia R, Coleman MP, Gloeckler Ries LA, Berrino F (2002). Childhood cancer survival in Europe and the United States. *Cancer*, **95**, 1767–72.

Gatta G, Capocaccia R, Stiller C *et al.* (2005). Childhood Cancer Survival Trends in Europe: a EURO-CARE Working Group Study. *Journal of Clinical Oncology*, **23**, 3742–51.

Gatta G, Corazziari I, Magnani C *et al.* (2003). Childhood cancer survival in Europe. *Annals of Oncology*, **14**, vl19–v127.

German Childhood Cancer Registry. (2002). German Childhood Cancer Registry Annual Report 2002 (1980–2001). Kaatsch, P. and Spix, C. Mainz, German Childhood Cancer Registry.

Gibson BES, Wheatley K, Hann IM *et al.* (2005). Treatment strategy and long-term results in paediatric patients treated in consecutive UK AML trials. *Leukemia*, **19**, 2130–8.

Gill M, Murrells T, McCarthy M, Silcocks P (1988). Chemotherapy for the primary treatment of osteosarcoma: population effectiveness over 20 years. *Lancet*, **1**, 689–92.

Gonzalez JR, Fernandez E, de Toledo JS *et al.* (2004). Trends in childhood cancer incidence and mortality in Catalonia, Spain, 1975–1998. *European Journal of Cancer Prevention*, **13**, 47–51.

Goodman MT, Gurney JG, Smith MA, Olshan AF (1999). Sympathetic nervous system tumours. In: Gloeckler Ries LA, Smith MA, Gurney JG, Linet M, Tamra T, Young JL, Bunin GR (eds.) *Cancer Incidence and Survival among Children and Adolescents: United States SEER Program 1975–1995*, NIH Pub No 99-4649, Bethesda, MD, pp. 65–72.

Goodwin RG, Holme SA, Roberts DL (2004). Variations in registration of skin cancer in the United Kingdom. *Clinical and Experimental Dermatology*, **29**, 328–30.

Goubin A, Auclerc MF, Auvrignon A *et al.* (2006). Survival in France after childhood acute leukaemia and non-Hodgkin's lymphoma (1990–2000). *European Journal of Cancer*, **42**, 534–41.

Gurney JG, Smith MA, Bunin GR (1999a). CNS and miscellaneous intracranial and intraspinal neoplasms. In: Gloeckler Ries LA, Smith MA, Gurney JG, Linet M, Tamra T, Young JL, Bunin GR (eds.) *Cancer Incidence and Survival among Children and Adolescents: United States SEER Program 1975–1995*, NIH Pub No 99–4649, Bethesda, MD, pp. 51–63.

Gurney JG, Smith MA, Ross JA (1999b). Cancer among infants. In: Gloeckler Ries LA, Smith MA, Gurney JG, Linet M, Tamra T, Young JL, Bunin GR (eds.) *Cancer Incidence and Survival among Children and Adolescents: United States SEER Program 1975–1995*, NIH Pub No 99–4649, Bethesda, MD, pp. 149–56.

Gurney JG, Swensen AR, Bulterys M (1999c). Malignant bone tumors. In: Gloeckler Ries LA, Smith MA, Gurney JG, Linet M, Tamra T, Young JL, Bunin GR (eds.) *Cancer Incidence and Survival among Children and Adolescents: United States SEER Program 1975–1995*, NIH Pub No 99–4649, Bethesda, MD, pp. 99–110.

Gurney JG, Wall DA, Jukich PJ, Davis FG (1999d). The contribution of nonmalignant tumors to CNS tumor incidence rates among children in the United States. *Cancer Causes & Control: CCC*, **10**, 101–5.

Gurney JG, Young JL, Roffers SD, Smith MA, Bunin GR (1999e). Soft tissue sarcomas. In: Gloeckler Ries LA, Smith MA, Gurney JG, Linet M, Tamra T, Young JL, Bunin GR (eds.) *Cancer Incidence and Survival among Children and Adolescents: United States SEER Program 1975–1995*, NIH Pub No 99–4649, Bethesda, MD, pp. 111–23.

Gustafsson G, Schmiegelow K, Forestier E *et al.* (2000). Improving outcome through two decades in childhood ALL in the Nordic countries: the impact of high-dose methotrexate in the reduction of CNS irradiation. *Leukemia*, **14**, 2267–75.

Hann IM, Eden OB, Barnes J, Pinkerton CR, on behalf of the United Kingdom Children's Cancer Study Group (UKCCSG) (1990). 'MACHO' chemotherapy for stage IV B cell lymphoma and B cell acute lymphoblastic leukaemia of childhood. *British Journal of Haematology*, **76**, 359–64.

Hann IM, Richards SM, Eden OB, Hill FGH, on behalf of the Medical Research Council Childhood Leukaemia Working Party (1998). Analysis of the immunophenotype of children treated on the Medical Research Council United Kingdom Acute Lymphoblastic Leukaemia Trial XI (MRC UKALLXI). *Leukemia*, **12**, 1249–55.

Hann IM, Stevens RF, Goldstone AH *et al.* (1997). Randomized comparison of DAT versus ADE as induction chemotherapy in children and younger adults with acute myeloid leukemia. Results of the Medical Research Council's 10th AML trial (MRC AML10). *Blood*, **89**, 2311–8.

Harach HR, Williams ED (1995). Childhood thyroid cancer in England and Wales. *British Journal of Cancer*, **72**, 777–83.

Hasle H, Kerndrup G, Jacobsen BB (1995). Childhood myelodysplastic syndrome in Denmark: incidence and predisposing conditions. *Leukemia*, **9**, 1569–72.

Hasle H, Wadsworth LD, Massing BG, McBride M, Schultz KR (1999). A population-based study of childhood myelodysplastic syndrome in British Columbia, Canada. *British Journal of Haematology*, **106**, 1027–32.

Hawkins MM (1989). Long-term survival and cure after childhood cancer. *Archives of Disease in Childhood*, **64**, 798–807.

Hawkins MM, Draper GJ, Kingston JE (1987). Incidence of second primary tumours among childhood cancer survivors. *British Journal of Cancer*, **56**, 339–47.

Hawkins MM, Kingston JE, Kinnier Wilson LM (1990). Late deaths after treatment for childhood cancer. *Archives of Disease in Childhood*, **65**, 1356–63.

Hawkins MM, Kinnier Wilson LM, Stovall MA *et al.* (1992). Epipodophyllotoxins, alkylating agents, and radiation and risk of secondary leukaemia after childhood cancer. *British Medical Journal*, **304**, 951–8.

Hawkins MM Smith RA (1989). Pregnancy outcomes in childhood cancer survivors: probable effects of abdominal irradiation. *International Journal of Cancer*, **43**, 399–402.

Hawkins MM, Smith RA, Curtice LJ (1988). Childhood cancer survivors and their offspring studied through a postal survey of general practitioners: preliminary results. *Journal of the Royal College of General Practitioners*, **38**, 102–5.

Hawkins MM, Swerdlow AJ (1992). Completeness of cancer and death follow-up obtained through the National Health Service Central Register for England and Wales. *British Journal of Cancer*, **66**, 408–13.

Hilden JM, Meerbaum S, Burger P *et al.* (2004). Central nervous system atypical teratoid/rhabdoid tumor: results of therapy in children enrolled in a registry. *Journal of Clinical Oncology*, **22**, 2877–84.

Hjalgrim LL, Rostgaard K, Schmiegelow K *et al.* (2003). Age- and sex-specific incidence of childhood leukaemia by immunophenotype in the Nordic countries. *Journal of the National Cancer Institute*, **95**, 1539–44.

Honjo S, Doran HE, Stiller CA *et al.* (2003). Neuroblastoma trends in Osaka, Japan, and Great Britain 1970–1994, in relation to screening. *International Journal of Cancer*, **103**, 538–43.

Innis MD (1972). Nephroblastoma: possible index cancer of childhood. *The Medical Journal of Australia*, **1**, 18–20.

Izarzugaza I, Steliarova-Foucher E, Carmen Martos M, Zivkovic S (2006). Non-Hodgkin lymphomas incidence and survival in European children and adolescents (1978–1997): report from the ACCIS project. *European Journal of Cancer*, **42**, 2050–63.

Jemal A, Devesa SS, Fears TR, Fraumeni JF (2000). Retinoblastoma incidence and sunlight exposure. *British Journal of Cancer*, **82**, 1875–8.

Jemal A, Murray T, Ward E *et al.* (2005). Cancer statistics, 2005. *CA: A Cancer Journal for Clinicians*, **55**, 10–30.

Jenkinson HC, Hawkins MM, Stiller CA, Winter DL, Marsden HB, Stevens MCG (2004). Long-term population-based risks of second malignant neoplasms after childhood cancer in Britain. *British Journal of Cancer*, **91**, 1905–10.

Joshi D, Anderson JR, Paidas C, Breneman J, Parham DM, Crist W (2004). Age is an independent prognostic factor in rhabdomyosarcoma: a report from the Soft Tissue Sarcoma Committee of the Children's Oncology Group. *Pediatric Blood & Cancer*, **42**, 64–73.

Kaatsch P, Rickert CH, Kühl J, Schüz J, Michaelis J (2001). Population-based epidemiologic data on brain tumors in German children. *Cancer*, **92**, 3155–64.

Kaatsch P, Steliarova-Foucher E, Crocetti E, Magnani C, Spix C, Zambon P (2006). Time trends of cancer incidence in European children (1978–1997): report from the ACCIS project. *European Journal of Cancer*, **42**, 1961–71.

Kardos G, Baumann I, Passmore SJ *et al.* (2003). Refractory anemia in childhood: a retrospective analysis of 67 patients with particular reference to monosomy 7. *Blood*, **102**, 1997–2003.

Kingston JE, Hawkins MM, Draper GJ, Marsden HB, Kinnier Wilson LM (1987). Patterns of multiple primary tumours in patients treated for cancer during childhood. *British Journal of Cancer*, **56**, 331–8.

Kingston JE, Hungerford JL, Madreperla SA, Plowman PN (1996). Results of combined chemotherapy and radiotherapy for advanced intraocular retinoblastoma. *Archives of Ophthalmology*, **114**, 1339–43.

Kinlen LJ, Dickson M, Stiller CA (1995). Childhood leukaemia and non-Hodgkin's lymphoma near large rural construction sites, with a comparison with Sellafield nuclear site. *British Medical Journal*, **310**, 763–8.

Kinlen LJ, Hudson CM, Stiller CA (1991). Contacts between adults as evidence for an infective origin of childhood leukaemia: an explanation for the excess near nuclear establishments in West Berkshire? *British Journal of Cancer*, **64**, 549–54.

Kinnier Wilson LM, Draper GJ (1974). Neuroblastoma, its natural history and prognosis: a study of 487 cases. *British Medical Journal*, **3**, 301–7.

Knox EG (2005a). Childhood cancers and atmospheric carcinogens. *Journal of Epidemiology and Community Health*, **59**, 101–5.

Knox EG (2005b). Oil combustion and childhood cancers. *Journal of Epidemiology and Community Health*, **59**, 755–60.

Knox EG (2006). Roads, railways, and childhood cancers. *Journal of Epidemiology and Community Health*, **60**, 136–41.

Knudson AG (1971). Mutation and cancer: statistical study of retinoblastoma. *Proceedings of National Academy of Sciences USA*, **68**, 820–3.

Kramarova E, Mann JR, Magnani C, Corraziari I, Berrino F (2001). Survival of children with malignant germ cell, trophoblastic and other gonadal tumours in Europe. *European Journal of Cancer*, **37**, 750–9.

Kramárová E, Stiller CA (1996). The international classification of childhood cancer. *International Journal of Cancer*, **68**, 759–65.

Kroll ME, Draper GJ, Stiller CA, Murphy MFG (2006). Childhood leukemia incidence in Britain, 1974–2000: time trends and possible relation to influenza epidemics. *Journal of the National Cancer Institute*, **98**, 417–20.

Kroll ME, Passmore SJ, Stiller CA et al. (2004). Chapter 9: Childhood Cancer – UK. *CancerStats Monograph 2004 – cancer incidence, survival and mortality in the UK and EU*, Cancer Research UK, 63–72.

Kunze U, Waldhoer T, Haidinger G (1997). Childhood cancer mortality in Austria, 1980–1992. *European Journal of Epidemiology*, **13**, 41–4.

La Vecchia C, Levi F, Lucchini F, Kaye SB, Boyle P (1991). Hodgkin's disease mortality in Europe. *British Journal of Cancer*, **64**, 723–34.

Lawson SE, Harrison G, Richards S et al. (2000). The UK experience in treating relapsed childhood acute lymphoblastic leukaemia: a report on the Medical Research Council UKALLR1 study. *British Journal of Haematology*, **108**, 531–43.

Leck I, Birch JM, Marsden HB, Steward JK (1976). Methods of classifying and ascertaining children's tumours. *British Journal of Cancer*, **34**, 69–82.

Legler JM, Gloeckler Ries LA, Smith MA et al. (1999). Brain and other central nervous system cancers: recent trends in incidence and mortality. *Journal of the National Cancer Institute*, **91**, 1382–90.

Leman JA, Evans A, Mooi W, MacKie RM (2005). Outcomes and pathological review of a cohort of children with melanoma. *The British Journal of Dermatology*, **152**, 1321–3.

Lennox EL, Stiller CA, Morris Jones PH, Kinnier Wilson LM (1979). Nephroblastoma: treatment during 1970–3 and the effect on survival of inclusion in the first MRC trial. *British Medical Journal*, **2**, 567–9.

Levi F, La Vecchia C (1988). Childhood cancer in Switzerland: Mortality from 1951 to 1984. *Oncology*, **45**, 313–7.

Levi F, La Vecchia C, Lucchini F, Negri E, Boyle P (1992). Patterns of childhood cancer incidence and mortality in Europe. *European Journal of Cancer*, **28A**, 2028–49.

Levi F, La Vecchia C, Negri E, Lucchini F (2001). Childhood cancer mortality in Europe, 1955–1995. *European Journal of Cancer*, **37**, 785–809.

Levi F, Lucchini F, Negri E, Barbui T, La Vecchia C (2000). Trends in mortality from leukemia in subsequent age groups. *Leukemia*, **14**, 1980–5.

Levitt G, Bunch KJ, Rogers CA, Whitehead B (1996). Cardiac transplantation in childhood cancer survivors in Britain. *European Journal of Cancer*, **32A**, 826–30.

Lie SO, Abrahamsson J, Clausen N *et al.* (2005). Long-term results in children with AML: NOPHO-AML Study Group – report of three consecutive trials. *Leukemia*, **19**, 2090–100.

Lie SO, Jonmundsson G, Mellander L *et al.* (1996). A population-based study of 272 children with acute myeloid leukaemia treated on two consecutive protocols with different intensity: best outcome in girls, infants, and children with Down's syndrome. *British Journal of Haematology*, **94**, 82–8.

Lightfoot T, Bunch K, Ansell P, Murphy M (2005). Ovulation induction, assisted conception and childhood cancer. *European Journal of Cancer*, **41**, 715–24.

Linet MS, Ries LAG, Smith MA, Tarone RE, Devesa SS (1999). Recent trends in childhood cancer incidence and mortality in the United States. *Journal of the National Cancer Institute*, **91**, 1051–8.

Little MP, Muirhead CR, Stiller CA (1996). Modelling lymphocytic leukaemia incidence in England and Wales using generalisations of the two-mutation model of carcinogenesis of Moolgavkar, Venzon and Knudson. *Statistics in Medicine*, **15**, 1003–22.

Lones MA, Auperin A, Raphael M *et al.* (2000). Mature B-cell lymphoma/leukemia in children and adolescents: intergroup pathologist consensus with the revised European–American Lymphoma Classification. *Annals of Oncology*, **11**, 47–51.

Lyons RA, Monaghan SP, Heaven M, Littlepage BNC, Vincent TJ, Draper GJ (1995). Incidence of leukaemia and lymphoma in young people in the vicinity of the petrochemical plant at Baglan Bay, South Wales, 1974–1991. *Occupational and Environmental Medicine*, **52**, 225–8.

MacCarthy A, Draper GJ, Steliarova-Foucher E, Kingston JE (2006). Retinoblastoma incidence and survival in European children (1978–1997): report from the ACCIS project. *European Journal of Cancer*, **42**, 2092–102.

Madreperla SA, Hungerford JL, Doughty D, Plowman PN, Kingston JE, Singh AD (1998). Treatment of retinoblastoma vitreous base seeding. *Ophthalmology*, **105**, 120–4.

Magnani C, Pastore G, Coebergh JWW, Viscomi S, Spix C, Steliarova-Foucher E (2006). Trends in survival after childhood cancer in Europe, 1978–97: report from the ACCIS project. *European Journal of Cancer*, **42**, 1981–2005.

Makepeace AR, MacLennan KA, Vaughan Hudson G, Jelliffe AM (1987). Hodgkin's disease in childhood: the British National Lymphoma Investigation experience (BNLI Report No 27). *Clinical Radiology*, **38**, 7–11.

Malec E, Lagerlof B (1977). Malignant melanoma of the skin in children registered in the Swedish cancer registry during 1959–1971. *Scandinavian Journal of Plastic and Reconstructive Surgery*, **11**, 125–9.

Mann JR, Kasthuri N, Raafat F *et al.* (1990). Malignant hepatic tumours in children: incidence, clinical features and aetiology. *Paediatric and Perinatal Epidemiology*, **4**, 276–89.

Mann JR, Pearson D, Barrett A, Raafat F, Barnes JM, Wallendszus KR (1989). Results of the United Kingdom Children's Cancer Study Group's malignant germ cell tumor studies. *Cancer*, **63**, 1657–67.

Martos MC, Olsen JH (1993). Childhood cancer mortality in the European Community, 1950–1989. *European Journal of Cancer*, **29A**, 1783–9.

Maurer HM, Gehan EA, Beltangady M *et al.* (1993). The Intergroup Rhabdomyosarcoma Study-II. *Cancer*, **71**, 1904–22.

McKinney PA, Parslow RC, Lane SA *et al.* (1998). Epidemiology of childhood brain tumours in Yorkshire, UK, 1974–95: geographical distribution and changing patterns of occurrence. *British Journal of Cancer*, **78**, 974–9.

McNally RJQ, Alexander FE, Bithell JF (2006). Space-time clustering of childhood cancer in Great Britain: a national study, 1969–1993. *International Journal of Cancer*, **118**, 2840–6.

McNally RJQ, Birch JM, Taylor GM, Eden OB (2000). Incidence of childhood precursor B-cell acute lymphoblastic leukaemia in north-west England. *Lancet*, **356**, 485–6.

McNally RJQ, Cairns DP, Eden OB, Kelsey AM, Taylor GM, Birch JM (2001a). Examination of temporal trends in the incidence of childhood leukaemias and lymphomas provides aetiological clues. *Leukemia*, **15**, 1612–8.

McNally RJQ, Kelsey AM, Cairns DP, Taylor GM, Eden OB, Birch JM (2001b). Temporal increases in the incidence of childhood solid tumors seen in Northwest England (1954–1998) are likely to be real. *Cancer*, **92**, 1967–76.

McNally RJQ, Roman E, Cartwright RA (1999). Leukemias and lymphomas: time trends in the UK, 1984–93. *Cancer Causes & Control: CCC*, **10**, 35–42.

McNally RJQ, Rowland D, Roman E, Cartwright RA (1997). Age and sex distributions of hematological malignancies in the UK. *Hematological Oncology*, **15**, 173–89.

McNeil DE, Coté TR, Clegg L, Rorke LB (2002). Incidence and trends in pediatric malignancies medulloblastoma/primitive neuroectodermal tumor: a SEER update. *Medical and Pediatric Oncology*, **39**, 190–4.

McWhirter WR, Dobson C (1995). Childhood melanoma in Australia. *World Journal of Surgery*, **19**, 334–6.

McWhirter WR, Dobson C, Ring I (1996). Childhood cancer incidence in Australia, 1982–1991. *International Journal of Cancer*, **65**, 34–8.

McWhirter WR, Stiller CA, Lennox EL (1989). Carcinomas in childhood. A registry-based study of incidence and survival. *Cancer*, **63**, 2242–6.

Medical Research Council working party on bone sarcoma (1986). A trial of chemotherapy in patients with osteosarcoma. (A report to the Medical Research Council by their Working Party on Bone Sarcoma). *British Journal of Cancer*, **53**, 513–8.

Medical Research Council's working party on embryonal tumours in Childhood (1978). Management of nephroblastoma in childhood. Clinical study of two forms of maintenance chemotherapy. *Archives of Disease in Childhood*, **53**, 112–9.

Medical Research Council's working party on leukaemia in childhood (1977). Treatment of acute lymphoblastic leukaemia: effect of variation in length of treatment on duration of remission. Report to the Medical Research Council by the Working Party on Leukaemia in Childhood. *British Medical Journal*, **2**, 495–7.

Menu-Branthomme A, Rubino C, Shamsaldin A *et al.* (2004). Radiation dose, chemotherapy and risk of soft tissue sarcoma after solid tumours during childhood. *International Journal of Cancer*, **110**, 87–93.

Mertens AC, Yasui Y, Neglia JP *et al.* (2001). Late mortality experience in five-year survivors of childhood and adolescent cancer: the Childhood Cancer Survivor Study. *Journal of Clinical Oncology*, **19**, 3163–72.

Michalkiewicz E, Sandrini R, Figueiredo B *et al.* (2004). Clinical and outcome characteristics of children with adrenocortical tumors: a report from the International Pediatric Adrenocortical Tumor Registry. *Journal of Clinical Oncology*, **22**, 838–45.

Mitchell C, Morris Jones P, Kelsey A *et al.* (2000). The treatment of Wilms' tumour: results of the United Kingdom Children's Cancer Study Group (UKCCSG) second Wilms' tumour study. *British Journal of Cancer*, **83**, 602–8.

Moll AC, Kuik DJ, Bouter LM *et al.* (1997). Incidence and survival of retinoblastoma in the Netherlands: a register-based study 1862–1995. *British Journal of Ophthalmology*, **81**, 559–62.

Möller TR, Garwicz S, Barlow L *et al.* (2001). Decreasing late mortality among five-year survivors of cancer in childhood and adolescence: a population-based study in the Nordic countries. *Journal of Clinical Oncology*, **19**, 3173–81.

Morton LM, Wang SS, Devesa SS, Hartge P, Weisenburger DD, Linet MS (2006). Lymphoma incidence patterns by WHO subtype in the United States, 1992–2001. *Blood*, **107**, 265–76.

Mott MG, Chessells JM, Willoughby MLN *et al.* (1984a). Adjuvant low-dose radiation in childhood T cell leukaemia/lymphoma. (Report from the United Kingdom Children's Cancer Study Group – UKCCSG). *British Journal of Cancer*, **50**, 457–62.

Mott MG, Eden OB, Palmer MK (1984b). Adjuvant low-dose radiation in childhood non-Hodgkin's lymphoma. (Report from the United Kingdom Children's Cancer Study Group – UKCCSG). *British Journal of Cancer*, **50**, 463–9.

Mott MG, Mann JR, Stiller CA (1997). The United Kingdom Children's Cancer Study Group – the first 20 years of growth and development. *European Journal of Cancer*, **33**, 1448–52.

Mueller BU (1999). Cancers in children infected with the human immunodeficiency virus. *The Oncologist*, **4**, 309–17.

Murphy MFG, Whiteman D, Hey K *et al.* (2001). Childhood cancer incidence in a cohort of twin babies. *British Journal of Cancer*, **84**, 1460–2.

Narod SA, Hawkins MM, Robertson CM, Stiller CA (1997). Congenital anomalies and childhood cancer in Great Britain. *American Journal of Human Genetics*, **60**, 474–85.

Neale RE, Mineau G, Whiteman DC, Brownbill PA, Murphy MFG (2005). Childhood and adult cancer in twins: evidence from the Utah genealogy. *Cancer Epidemiology Biomarkers and Prevention*, **14**, 1236–40.

Netherlands Cancer Registry (2000). Childhood cancer in the Netherlands 1989–1997. Coebergh JWW, van Dijk JAAM, Janssen-Heijnen MLG, Visser O, Association of Comprehensive Cancer Centres, Utrecht, Netherlands.

Newnham A, Møller H (2002). Trends in the incidence of cutaneous malignant melanomas in the south east of England, 1960–1998. *J Public Health Med*, **24**, 268–75.

Niemeyer CM, Aricó M, Basso G *et al.* (1997). Chronic myelomonocytic leukemia in childhood: a retrospective analysis of 110 cases. *Blood*, **89**, 3534–43.

Owen PJ, Miles DPB, Draper GJ, Vincent TJ (2002). Retrospective study of mortality after a water pollution incident at Lowermoor in north Cornwall. *British Medical Journal*, **324**, 1189.

Parkes SE, Muir KR, Al Sheyyab M *et al.* (1993). Carcinoid tumours of the appendix in children 1957–1986: incidence, treatment and outcome. *British Journal of Surgery*, **80**, 502–4.

Parkes SE, Muir KR, Camerson AH *et al.* (1997). The need for specialist review of pathology in paediatric cancer. *British Journal of Cancer*, **75**, 1156–9.

Parkin DM, Cardis E, Masuyer E *et al.* (1993). Childhood leukaemia following the Chernobyl accident: The European Childhood Leukaemia–Lymphoma Incidence Study (ECLIS). *European Journal of Cancer*, **29A**, 87–95.

Parkin DM, Whelan SL, Ferlay J, Teppo L, Thomas DB (eds.) (2002) *Cancer Incidence in Five Continents Volume VIII*, IARC Scientific Publications No. 155, IARC, Lyon.

Parkin DM, Kramárová E, Draper GJ, Masuyer E, Michaelis J, Neglia J, Qureshi S, Stiller CA (eds.) (1998) *International Incidence of Childhood Cancer: Volume 2*, IARC, Lyon.

Parkin DM, Stiller CA, Draper GJ, Bieber CA (1988a). The international incidence of childhood cancer. *International Journal of Cancer*, **42**, 511–20.

Parkin DM, Stiller CA, Draper GJ, Bieber CA, Terracini B, Young JL (eds.) (1988b). *International Incidence of Childhood Cancer (IARC Scientific Publications No. 87)*. International Agency for Research on Cancer, Lyon.

Partoft S, Østerlind A, Hou-Jensen K, Drzewiecki KT (1989). Malignant melanoma of the skin in children (0 to 14 years of age) in Denmark, 1943–1982. *Scandinavian Journal of Plastic and Reconstructive Surgery*, **23**, 55–8.

Passmore SJ, Chessells JM, Kempski H, Hann IM, Brownbill PA, Stiller CA (2003). Paediatric myelodysplastic syndromes and juvenile myelomonocytic leukaemia in the UK: a population-based study of incidence and survival. *British Journal of Haematology*, **121**, 758–67.

Passmore SJ, Draper GJ, Brownbill PA, Kroll ME (1998a). Case-control studies of relation between childhood cancer and neonatal vitamin K administration. *British Medical Journal*, **316**, 178–84.

Passmore SJ, Draper GJ, Brownbill PA, Kroll ME (1998b). Ecological studies of relation between hospital policies on neonatal vitamin K administration and subsequent occurrence of childhood cancer. *British Medical Journal*, **316**, 184–9.

Pastore G, Peris-Bonet R, Carli M, Martíinez-García C, Sánchez de Toledo J, Steliarova-Foucher E (2006a). Childhood soft tissue sarcomas. Incidence and survival in European children (1978–97): report from ACCIS project. *European Journal of Cancer*, **42**, 2136–49.

Pastore G, Znaor A, Spreafico F, Graf N, Pritchard-Jones K, Steliarova-Foucher E (2006b). Malignant renal tumours incidence and survival in European children (1978–1997): report from the ACCIS project. *European Journal of Cancer*, **42**, 2103–14.

Pearce MS, Parker L, Cotterill SJ, Gordon PM, Craft AW (2003). Skin cancer in children and young adults: 28 years' experience from the Northern Region Young Person's Malignant Disease Registry, UK. *Melanoma Res*, **13**, 421–6.

Pearce MS, Parker L, Windebank KP, Cotterill SJ, Craft AW (2005). Cancer in adolescents and young adults aged 15–24 years: a report from the North of England Young Person's Malignant Disease Registry, UK. *Pediatric Blood & Cancer*, **45**, 687–93.

Pearson ADJ, Pinkerton CR, Lewis IJ (1994). European Neuroblastoma Group Fifth Study (ENSG 5). A randomised study of dose intensity in stage 4 neuroblastoma over the age of one. In: Evans AE, Biedler JL, Brodeur GM, D'Angio GJ, Nakagawara A (eds.) *Progress in Clinical and Biological Research – Advances in Neuroblastoma Research*, Wiley-Liss, New York, 385–94.

Percy CL, Smith MA, Linet M, Gloeckler Ries LA, Friedman DL (1999). Lymphomas and reticuloen-dothelial neoplasms. In: Gloeckler Ries LA, Smith MA, Gurney JG, Linet M, Tamra T, Young JL, Bunin GR (eds.) *Cancer Incidence and Survival among Children and Adolescents: United States SEER Program 1975–1995*, NIH Pub No 99–4649, Bethesda, MD, pp. 35–49.

Peris-Bonet R, Martínez-García C, Lacour B *et al.* (2006). Childhood central nervous system tumours. Incidence and survival in Europe (1978–1997): report from the ACCIS project. *European Journal of Cancer*, **42**, 2064–80.

Perkins JL, Liu Y, Mitby PA *et al.* (2005). Nonmelanoma skin cancer in survivors of childhood and adolescent cancer: a report from the childhood cancer survivor study. *Journal of Clinical Oncology*, **23**, 3733–41.

Peto R, Pike MC, Armitage P *et al.* (1977). Design and analysis of randomized clinical trials requiring prolonged observation of each patient. II. Analysis and examples. *British Journal of Cancer*, **35**, 1–39.

Pinkerton CR, Hann I, Eden OB *et al.* (1991). Outcome in stage III non-Hodgkin's lymphoma in children (UKCCSG study NHL 86) – How much treatment is needed? *British Journal of Cancer*, **64**, 583–7.

Pizer BL, Weston CL, Robinson KJ *et al.* (2006). Analysis of patients with supratentorial primitive neuro-ectodermal tumours entered into the SIOP/UKCCSG PNET 3 study. *European Journal of Cancer*, **42**, 1120–8.

Powell JE, Esteve J, Mann JR *et al.* (1998). Neuroblastoma in Europe: differences in the pattern of disease in the UK. *Lancet*, **352**, 682–7.

Pritchard J, Brown J, Shafford E *et al.* (2000). Cisplatin, doxorubicin, and delayed surgery for childhood hepatoblastoma: a successful approach – results of the first prospective study of the International Society of Pediatric Oncology. *Journal of Clinical Oncology*, **18**, 3819–28.

Pritchard J, Cotterill SJ, Germond SM, Imeson J, de Kraker J, Jones DR (2005). High-dose Melphalan in the treatment of advanced neuroblastoma: results of a randomised trial (ENSG-1) by the European Neuroblastoma Study Group. *Pediatric Blood & Cancer*, **44**, 348–57.

Pritchard J, Imeson J, Barnes J *et al.* (1995). Results of the United Kingdom Children's Cancer Study Group first Wilms' tumor study. *Journal of Clinical Oncology*, **13**, 124–33.

Pritchard J, Stiller CA, Lennox EL (1989). Over-treatment of children with Wilms' tumour outside paediatric oncology centres. *British Medical Journal*, **299**, 835–6.

Punyko JA, Mertens AC, Scott Baker K, Ness KK, Robison LL, Gurney JG (2005). Long-term survival probabilities for childhood rhabdomyosarcoma. A population-based evaluation. *Cancer*, **103**, 1475–83.

Rao A, Hills RK, Stiller C et al. (2006). Treatment for myeloid leukaemia of Down syndrome: population-based experience in the UK and results from the Medical Research Council AML 10 and AML 12 trials. *British Journal of Haematology*, **132**, 576–83.

Richardson S, Monfort C, Green M, Draper GJ, Muirhead C (1995). Spatial variation of natural radiation and childhood leukaemia incidence in Great Britain. *Statistics in Medicine*, **14**, 2487–501.

Ries LAG, Harkins D, Krapcho M, Mariotto A, Miller BA, Feuer EJ, Clegg L, Eisner MP, Horner MJ, Howlader N, Hayat M, Hankey BF, Edwards BK (eds.) (2006) *SEER Cancer Statistics Review, 1975–2003*. National Cancer Institute, Bethesda, MD.

Ries LAG, Smith MA, Gurney JG, Linet M, Tamra T, Young JL, Bunin GR (eds.) (1999) *Cancer Incidence and Survival among Children and Adolescents: United States SEER Program 1975–1995*, National Cancer Institute SEER Program. NIH Pub No 99-4649. Bethesda, MD.

Riley LC, Hann IM, Wheatley K, Stevens RF (1999). Treatment-related deaths during induction and first remission of acute myeloid leukaemia in children treated on the Tenth Medical Research Council acute myeloid leukaemia trial (MRC AML10). *British Journal of Haematology*, **106**, 436–44.

Robertson CM and Hawkins MM (1995). Childhood cancer and cystic fibrosis (corres). *Journal of the National Cancer Institute*, **87**, 1486–7.

Robertson CM, Hawkins MM, Kingston JE (1994). Late deaths and survival after childhood cancer: implications for cure. *British Medical Journal*, **309**, 162–6.

Robertson CM, Stiller CA, Kingston JE (1992). Causes of death in children diagnosed with non-Hodgkin's lymphoma between 1974 and 1985. *Archives of Disease in Childhood*, **67**, 1378–83.

Robison LL, Green DM, Hudson M et al. (2005). Long-term outcomes of adult survivors of childhood cancer. Results from the Childhood Cancer Survivor Study. *Cancer*, **104**, 2557–64.

Robison LL, Mertens AC, Boice JD et al. (2002). Study design and cohort characteristics of the Childhood Cancer Survivor Study: a multi-institutional collaborative project. *Medical and Pediatric Oncology*, **38**, 229–39.

Saksela E, Rintala A (1968). Misdiagnosis of prepubertal malignant melanoma. Reclassification of a cancer registry material. *Cancer*, **22**, 1308–14.

Sanders BM, Draper GJ, Kingston JE (1988). Retinoblastoma in Great Britain 1969–80: incidence, treatment, and survival. *British Journal of Ophthalmology*, **72**, 576–83.

Sankila R, Martos Jiménez MC, Miljus D, Pritchard-Jones K, Steliarova-Foucher E, Stiller C (2006). Geographical comparison of cancer survival in European children (1988–1997): report from the ACCIS project. *European Journal of Cancer*, **42**, 1972–80.

Satgé D, Sasco AJ, Carlsen NLT et al. (1998). A lack of neuroblastoma in Down Syndrome: a study from 11 European countries. *Cancer Research*, **58**, 448–52.

Schilling FH, Spix C, Berthold F et al. (2002). Neuroblastoma screening at one year of age. *New England Journal of Medicine*, **346**, 1047–53.

Schrappe M, Reiter A, Zimmermann M et al. (2000). Long-term results of four consecutive trials in childhood ALL performed by the ALL–BFM study group from 1981 to 1995. *Leukemia*, **14**, 2205–22.

Shah A (2005). Childhood leukaemia in Great Britain: trends in incidence, survival and 'cure' (Thesis). Non-Communicable Disease Epidemiology Unit, London School of Hygiene and Tropical Medicine, pp. 1–269.

Shankar AG, Ashley S, Radford M, Barrett A, Wright D, Pinkerton CR (1997). Does histology influence outcome in childhood Hodgkin's disease? Results from the United Kingdom Children's Cancer Study Group. *Journal of Clinical Oncology*, **15**, 2622–30.

Shapiro NL, Bhattacharyya N (2005). Population-based outcomes for pediatric thyroid carcinoma. *Laryngoscope*, **115**, 337–40.

Shibata Y, Yamashita S, Masayakin VB, Panasyuk GD, Nagataki S (2001). 15 years after Chernobyl: new evidence of thyroid cancer. *Lancet*, **358**, 1965–6.

Smith MA, Freidlin B, Gloeckler Ries LA, Simon R (1998). Trends in reported incidence of primary malignant brain tumors in children in the United States. *Journal of the National Cancer Institute*, **90**, 1269–77.

Smith MA, Gloeckler Ries LA, Gurney JG, Ross JA (1999a). Leukaemia. In: Gloeckler Ries LA, Smith MA, Gurney JG, Linet M, Tamra T, Young JL, Bunin GR (eds.) *Cancer Incidence and Survival among Children and Adolescents: United States SEER Program 1975–1995*, NIH Pub No 99-4649, Bethesda, MD, pp. 17–34.

Smith MA, Gurney JG, Gloeckler Ries LA (1999b). Cancer among adolescents 15–19 years old. In: Gloeckler Ries LA, Smith MA, Gurney JG, Linet M, Tamra T, Young JL, Bunin GR (eds.) *Cancer Incidence and Survival among Children and Adolescents: United States SEER Program 1975–1995*, NIH Pub No 99-4649, Bethesda, MD, pp. 157–64.

Sorahan T, Haylock RGE, Muirhead CR *et al.* (2003). Cancer in the offspring of radiation workers: an investigation of employment timing and a reanalysis using updated dose information. *British Journal of Cancer*, **89**, 1215–20.

Spix C, Pastore G, Sankila R, Stiller CA, Steliarova-Foucher E (2006). Neuroblastoma incidence and survival in European children (1978–1997): report from the ACCIS project. *European Journal of Cancer*, **42**, 2081–91.

Stang A, Streller B, Katalinic A *et al.* (2006). Incidence of skin lymphoma in Germany. *Annals of Epidemiology*, **16**, 214–22.

Stansfeld AG, Diebold J, Kapanci Y *et al.* (1988). Updated Kiel classification for lymphomas (corres.). *Lancet*, **1**, 292–3.

Steliarova-Foucher E, Kaatsch P, Lacour B *et al.* (2006a). Quality, comparability and methods of analysis of data on childhood cancer in Europe (1978–1997): report from the ACCIS project. *European Journal of Cancer*, **42**, 1915–51.

Steliarova-Foucher E, Stiller C, Kaatsch P *et al.* (2004). Geographical patterns and time trends of cancer incidence and survival among children and adolescents in Europe since the 1970s (the ACCIS project): an epidemiological study. *Lancet*, **364**, 2097–105.

Steliarova-Foucher E, Stiller C, Kaatsch P, Berrino F, Coebergh JW (2005a). Trends in childhood cancer incidence in Europe, 1970–99. *Lancet*, **365**, 2088.

Steliarova-Foucher E, Stiller C, Lacour B, Kaatsch P (2005b). International classification of childhood cancer, third edition. *Cancer*, **103**, 1457–67.

Steliarova-Foucher E, Stiller CA, Pukkala E, Lacour B, Plesko I, Parkin DM (2006b). Thyroid cancer incidence and survival among European children and adolescents (1978–97) project. Report from the ACCIS. *European Journal of Cancer*, **42**, 2150–69.

Stevens MCG (2006). The 'Lost Tribe' and the need for a promised land: the challenge of cancer in teenagers and young adults. *European Journal of Cancer*, **42**, 280–1.

Stevens MCG, Rey A, Bouvet N *et al.* (2005). Treatment of nonmetastatic rhabdomyosarcoma in childhood and adolescence: third study of the International Society of Paediatric Oncology – SIOP Malignant Mesenchymal Tumor 89. *Journal of Clinical Oncology*, **23**, 2618–28.

Stevens RF, Hann IM, Wheatley K, Gray RG, on behalf of the MRC Childhood Leukaemia Working Party (1998). Marked improvements in outcome with chemotherapy alone in paediatric acute myeloid leukaemia: results of the United Kingdom Medical Research Council's 10th AML trial. *British Journal of Haematology*, **101**, 130–40.

Stewart A, Webb J, Hewitt D (1958). A survey of childhood malignancies. *British Medical Journal*, **30**, 1495–508.

Stiller CA (1988). Centralisation of treatment and survival rates for cancer. *Archives of Disease in Childhood*, **63**, 23–30.

Stiller CA (1994a). Centralised treatment, entry to trials and survival. *British Journal of Cancer*, **70**, 352–62.

Stiller CA (1994b). International variations in the incidence of childhood carcinomas. *Cancer Epidemiology Biomarkers and Prevention*, 3, 305–10.

Stiller CA, Allen MB, Eatock EM (1995). Childhood cancer in Britain; The national registry of childhood tumours and incidence rates 1978–1987. *European Journal of Cancer*, 31, 2028–34.

Stiller CA, Benjamin S, Cartwright RA *et al.* (1999). Patterns of care and survival for adolescents and young adults with acute leukaemia – a population-based study. *British Journal of Cancer*, 79, 658–65.

Stiller CA, Bielack SS, Jundt G, Steliarova-Foucher E (2006a). Bone tumours in European children and adolescents, 1978–1997. Report from the ACCIS project. *European Journal of Cancer*, 42, 2124–35.

Stiller CA, Boyle PJ (1996). Effect of population mixing and socioeconomic status in England and Wales, 1979–85, on lymphoblastic leukaemia in children. *British Medical Journal*, 313, 1297–300.

Stiller CA, Bunch KJ, Lewis IJ (2000). Ethnic group and survival from childhood cancer: report from the UK Children's Cancer Study Group. *British Journal of Cancer*, 82, 1339–43.

Stiller CA, Chessells JM, Fitchett M (1994). Neurofibromatosis and childhood leukaemia/lymphoma: a population-based UKCCSG study. *British Journal of Cancer*, 70, 969–72.

Stiller CA, Draper GJ (1989). Treatment centre size, entry to trials, and survival in acute lymphoblastic leukaemia. *Archives of Disease in Childhood*, 64, 657–61.

Stiller CA, Eatock EM (1994). Survival from acute non-lymphocytic leukaemia, 1971–88: a population-based study. *Archives of Disease in Childhood*, 70, 219–23.

Stiller CA, Eatock EM (1999). Patterns of care and survival for children with acute lymphoblastic leukaemia diagnosed between 1980–94. *Archives of Disease in Childhood*, 81, 202–8.

Stiller CA, Marcos-Gragera R, Ardanaz E *et al.* (2006b). Geographical patterns of childhood cancer incidence in Europe, 1988–1997: report from the ACCIS project. *European Journal of Cancer*, 42, 1952–60.

Stiller CA, McKinney PA, Bunch KJ, Bailey CC, Lewis IJ (1991a). Childhood cancer and ethnic group in Britain: a United Kingdom Children's Cancer Study Group (UKCCSG) study. *British Journal of Cancer*, 64, 543–8.

Stiller CA, O'Connor CM, Vincent TJ, Draper GJ (1991b). The National Registry of Childhood Tumours and the leukaemia/lymphoma data for 1966–83. In: Draper GJ (ed.) *The Geographical Epidemiology of Childhood Leukaemia and Non-Hodgkin Lymphomas in Great Britain*, 1966–83, OPCS Studies on Medical and Population Subjects No. 53, HMSO, London, pp. 7–16.

Stiller CA, Parkin DM (1990). International variations in the incidence of childhood renal tumours. *British Journal of Cancer*, 62, 1026–30.

Stiller CA, Parkin DM (1996). Geographic and ethnic variations in the incidence of childhood cancer. *British Medical Bulletin*, 52, 682–703.

Stiller CA, Passmore SJ, Kroll ME, Brownbill PA, Wallis JC, Craft AW (2006c). Patterns of care and survival for patients aged under 40 years with bone sarcoma in Britain, 1980–1994. *British Journal of Cancer*, 94, 22–9.

Stiller CA, Pritchard J, Steliarova-Foucher E (2006d). Liver cancer in European children: incidence and survival, 1978–1997. Report from the ACCIS project. *European Journal of Cancer*, 42, 2115–23.

Strouse JJ, Fears TR, Tucker MA, Wayne AS (2005). Pediatric melanoma: risk factor and survival analysis of the Surveillance, Epidemiology and End Results database. *Journal of Clinical Oncology*, 23, 4735–41.

Swiss Childhood Cancer Registry (2005). Swiss Childhood Cancer Registry Annual Report 2004. Kuehni, C. Bern, Switzerland, Swiss Childhood Cancer Registry.

Tait DM, Thornton-Jones H, Bloom HJG, Lemerle J, Morris-Jones P (1990). Adjuvant chemotherapy for medulloblastoma: the first multi-centre control trial of the International Society of Paediatric Oncology (SIOP I). *European Journal of Cancer*, 26, 464–9.

Taylor A, Hawkins M, Griffiths A *et al.* (2004). Long-term follow-up of survivors of childhood cancer in the UK. *Pediatric Blood & Cancer*, 42, 161–8.

Taylor RE, Bailey CC, Robinson K *et al.* (2003). Results of a randomized study of preradiation chemotherapy versus radiotherapy alone for nonmetastatic medulloblastoma: the International Society of Paediatric Oncology/United Kingdom Children's Cancer Study Group PNET-3 Study. *Journal of Clinical Oncology*, **21**, 1581–91.

The Medical Research Council (1986). Improvement in treatment for children with acute lymphoblastic leukaemia The Medical Research Council UKALL Trials, 1972–84. *Lancet*, **1**, 408–11.

Tomlinson GE, Breslow NE, Dome J *et al.* (2005). Rhabdoid tumor of the kidney in the National Wilms' Tumor Study: age at diagnosis as a prognostic factor. *Journal of Clinical Oncology*, **23**, 7641–5.

UKCCSG (2002). Ablett S (ed.) *Quest for Cure: UK Children's Cancer Study Group – The First 25 Years.* Trident Communications Ltd., Leicester.

Valery PC, McWhirter W, Sleigh A, Williams G, Bain C (2002). Farm exposures, parental occupation, and risk of Ewing's sarcoma in Australia: a national case-control study. *Cancer Causes & Control: CCC*, **13**, 263–70.

Verrill MW, Judson IR, Harmer CL, Fisher C, Thomas JM, Wiltshaw E (1997). Ewing's sarcoma and primitive neuroectodermal tumor in adults: are they different from Ewing's sarcoma and primitive neuroectodermal tumor in children? *Journal of Clinical Oncology*, **15**, 2611–21.

Viscomi S, Pastore G, Mosso ML *et al.* (2003). Population-based analysis of survival after childhood cancer diagnosed during 1970–1998: a report from the Childhood Cancer Registry of Piedmont, Italy. *Haematologica*, **88**, 974–82.

Wabinga HR, Parkin DM, Wabwire-Mangen F, Nambooze S (2000). Trends in cancer incidence in Kyadondo county, Uganda, 1960–1997. *British Journal of Cancer*, **82**, 1585–92.

Walker DA, Grundy R, Stiller C (2002). Rare Tumours of Childhood. In: Souhami RL, Tannock I, Hohenberger P, Horoit J-C (eds.) *Oxford Textbook of Oncology Volume 2*, 2nd edn, Oxford University Press, Oxford, pp. 2669–91.

Weeks DA, Beckwith JB, Mierau GW, Luckey DW (1989). Rhabdoid tumor of kidney. A report of 111 cases from the National Wilms' Tumor Study Pathology Center. *The American Journal of Surgical Pathology*, **13**, 439–58.

Wilkinson JR, Feltbower RG, Lewis IJ, Parslow RC, McKinney PA (2001). Survival from adolescent cancer in Yorkshire, UK. *European Journal of Cancer*, **37**, 903–11.

World Health Organisation (2000). Fritz A, Percy C, Jack A, Shanmugaratnam K, Sobin L, Parkin DM, Whelan S (eds.) *International Classification of Diseases for Oncology*, 3rd Edition. WHO, Geneva.

World Health Organization (1976). *International Classification of Diseases for Oncology, ICD-O*. World Health Organization, Geneva.

World Health Organization (1990). Percy C, Van Holten V, Muir C (eds.) *International Classification of Diseases for Oncology Second Edition*. World Health Organization, Geneva.

World Health Organization (2001). Jaffe ES, Harris NL, Stein H, Vardiman JW (eds.) *Pathology and Genetics of Tumours of Haematopoietic and Lymphoid Tissues*. IARC Press, Lyon.

Wright D, McKeever P, Carter R (1997). Childhood non-Hodgkin lymphomas in the United Kingdom: findings from the UK Children's Cancer Study Group. *Journal of Clinical Pathology*, **50**, 128–34.

Young JL and Miller RW (1975). Incidence of malignant tumors in U.S. children. *Journal of Pediatrics*, **86**, 254–8.

Young JL, Smith MA, Roffers SD, Liff JM, Bunin GR (1999). Retinoblastoma. In: Gloeckler Ries LA, Smith MA, Gurney JG, Linet M, Tamra T, Young JL, Bunin GR (eds.) *Cancer Incidence and Survival among Children and Adolescents: United States SEER Program 1975–1995*, NIH Pub No 99-4649, Bethesda, MD, pp. 73–8.

Zuccolo L, Pastore G, Maule M *et al.* (2004). Time trends of childhood cancer mortality rates: A report from the Childhood Cancer Registry of Piedmont, Italy, 1971–1998. *Pediatric Blood & Cancer*, **43**, 796–9.

Index